THE TRUTH ABOUT TRANSPLANTS

The Truth About Transplants

Paulette Pratt

JANUS PUBLISHING COMPANY
London, England

First published in Great Britain 2012
by Janus Publishing Company Ltd,
93–95 Gloucester Place,
London W1U 6JQ

www.januspublishing.co.uk

British Library Cataloguing-in-Publication Data
A catalogue record for this book is available from the British Library

ISBN 978-1-85756-743-4

Cover Design: Baker
www.jackets.moonfruit.com

Printed and bound in Great Britain

Acknowledgements

This book draws together more than twenty years' experience developing the Gift of Life series of booklets published by the British Organ Donor Society (BODY). It is dedicated to the society's original trustees and to the many donor and recipient families and clinical staff who have been so generous with their time and thoughts. Thanks are due in particular to long-suffering verifiers: Sarah Beale, specialist nurse in organ donation, Oxford; Mr Bimbi Fernando, consultant surgeon at the Royal Free Hospital; Dame Julia Polak, Emeritus Professor of Imperial College; Mr Chris Rudge, consultant transplant surgeon and National Clinical Director for Transplantation; Emma Thirlwall, specialist nurse in organ donation; and John Wallwork, Professor of Cardiothoracic Surgery, Papworth Hospital.

‘The transplantation of organs will be assimilated into ordinary clinical practice ... This will come about for the single and sufficient reason that people are so constituted that they would rather be alive than dead.’

Sir Peter Medawar, addressing the Second International Congress of the Transplantation Society, New York City, 11th Septemeber 1968.

‘The growth of transplantation from ground zero to its present state seems like a fairy tale, a fantasy that became reality because of the courage of our patients. The truth is that none of us in the 1950s remotely envisioned the height to which transplantation would rise and the way it has changed the face of medicine.’

Transplant surgeon *Thomas Starzl*, quoted in a *New York Times* feature celebrating the 50th anniversary of the world’s first successful organ transplant, December 2004.

‘A dead brain in a body with a still beating heart is one of the more macabre products of modern technology.’

Opening sentence in the first edition of the ‘*ABC of Brainstem Death*’ by *Drs Christopher Pallis* and *David Hardy*.

‘One of the greatest things to come out of the Taskforce report for me has been the opportunity to see how much comfort families can receive from their loved ones becoming donors. It is those familites who need to be recognised and appreciated.’

Comment from *Elisabeth Buggins*, chair of the Organ Donation Taskforce, reported in the *UK Transplant’s* spring 2008 bulletin.

Foreword

This is the book that I wish I'd written – but it's far better for having been written by an extremely well-informed outsider than by someone who has spent almost all his professional life intimately involved with the miracle of modern medicine that is organ transplantation.

Transplantation fascinated me in the 1960s, when it was really struggling to prove that it was an acceptable and successful form of treatment for patients who would otherwise die, and it fascinates me still. This is because it poses an almost unparalleled range of challenges, from the astonishing developments of 21st-century science to age-old questions about what it is to be human, and of course what we understand by death.

For one person to receive a transplant of a human organ another human has to donate the organ – either in life (as a living donor) or after their death. Transplantation stretches the boundaries way beyond the simple concept of one doctor treating one patient, with drugs or surgery or however, because a donor is needed. Not only that, but if organs are to be donated after death they must be removed very soon after the donor has died, which means that we must be more certain than ever that we can say exactly when death has occurred. This immediately takes the whole subject into the realms of ethics, philosophy, law – and means that the subject rightly exists in a much wider, public, context than does much of medicine.

Paulette Pratt has titled her Introduction 'A dearth of information'. I admit to being slightly irritated when I first read this – surely there's a plethora of leaflets, booklets, websites and so-on on that are available to patients? But what has been missing – and what this book provides – is the story, as seen by the layman, of the way in which transplantation has developed, of the challenges that have been (and still are) faced, how these challenges are being tackled today and of how the whole organ donation and transplantation system actually works.

The book does not shirk the difficult and at times controversial aspects of transplantation. Over 8,000 people are currently waiting for a transplant, and on average three people die every day because the transplant they need does not become available. These deaths are avoidable, not inevitable, and the search for solutions will inevitably push at the boundaries. The book has understood this and gives a sympathetic but realistic appraisal of the situation in terms that everyone can understand. I very much enjoyed reading it.

Chris Rudge FRCS
National Clinical Director for Transplantation
June 2011

Contents

Introduction

A Dearth of Information

One of the most far-reaching developments in hospital medicine in recent years has been the attempt by the last government to take the whole business of organ transplantation by the scruff and try and sort it out. The rationale for this was provided by a specially convened organisation called the Organ Donation Taskforce, which published its report ('Organs for Transplants') in January 2008. It found many irregularities and came up with fourteen recommendations for putting it right, with the expectation that these changes would bring about a 50 per cent increase in organ donation rates over the ensuing five years.

The organs used for donation come from three sources: heartbeating donors; non-heartbeating donors; and, increasingly, living relatives or friends. Of course, there are relatively few people who either could or would surrender all or part of an organ in life and so the need for cadaver donors will continue to increase. In principle, a single donor can contribute eight solid organs: two kidneys, two lungs, a liver, heart, pancreas and small bowel; although this rarely, if ever, happens. Also, there are the other tissues: corneas, skin, bone, heart valves, cartilage and so on. As one hospital policy document says, 'The tissues donated by one donor may enable up to 40 people to benefit from tissue transplant surgery.'

Cadaver donation puts families in an extraordinary situation. Imagine what it must be like to be summoned to a major hospital, one which may be unfamiliar, to find a friend or relative dead or dying, and then to be asked if their organs can be removed for what amounts to recycling. This is possibly one of the most harrowing situations imaginable and yet there is a dearth of information to which people can turn. The NHS Blood and Transplant (NHSBT) website gives a few brief answers on donation in its Q & A section. Under the heading Donor Care, the reader is referred to five technical documents, including a chapter from the Intensive Care Society's guidelines for organ donor management, which can hardly be said to be user-friendly for bereaved people seeking to come to terms with loss.

There is very little on the NHSBT website on non-heartbeating donation and nothing at all on the retrieval surgery (the term 'harvesting', sometimes heard in the US, is frowned upon in this country). Yet a number of studies have shown that many bereaved relatives want to know exactly what happens to potential donors. Some even want to see diagrams and X-rays or scans to help them grasp what is taking place.

In practice, it is the responsibility of the donor transplant co-ordinators (recently renamed specialist nurses in organ donation, SNODs) to explain what is happening and many doctors and nurses working in critical care areas are also very good in this respect. However, bereaved people are in shock at the time they encounter clinical staff and so it is hard for them to absorb a mass of new information at this time. One of the SNODs is always there to reinforce information where necessary, both before and for some considerable time after the event, but there is a clear case to be made for supplying written and other material for the general public.

On the recipient side there is a wealth of information, although relatively few sources tackle the downside of transplantation: the fact that patients undergoing organ transplants exchange one set of problems for another. True, transplants are mostly life-saving or at the very least they offer a much improved quality of life but, while most recipients do very well, others face significant difficulties. All recipients live with the constant fear of infection, rejection or transplant-associated cancer.

There are some awkward truths to be faced in transplantation – all the way from the occasional wasted organs to the intransigence of some surgeons. Anyone familiar with the field can hardly fail to be amused by a couple of paragraphs in a later report by Elisabeth Buggins, Chair of the Organ Donation Taskforce. She observes that most pioneering areas of medicine seem to attract 'strong characters': 'Whilst these individuals can put relationships with colleagues, management and other transplant centres under strain, it should not be forgotten that patients may benefit from their determined and driven nature, their willingness to take risks for their patient's benefit and their supreme technical skill ...

'However if the actions of these strong characters damage public confidence in the organ donor system, resulting in a significant fall in donor organs from an already low base, they may cause more harm than good.'

All along, the drive to donate has been affected by publicity. Older members of the transplant community still shudder to recall the effect of the notorious *Panorama* programme *'Are the donors really dead?'*, which, transmitted in October 1980, questioned the validity of the brainstem death diagnosis. In the four weeks following the transmission, kidney transplants fell by a quarter. It has to be said that the question posed in the programme's title still lingers in the minds of some people.

Organ donation received a sustained boost four years later from the Ben Hardwick story taken up by Esther Rantzen and the *That's Life* team. Ben was a toddler born with biliary atresia, a congenital condition in which the ducts draining bile from the liver are blocked or missing. A leading transplant surgeon urged the toddler's mother to 'mobilise public opinion' and this is exactly what she did, in what is believed to have been the first TV appeal for an organ. As a result a liver was found, enabling Ben to become the first child in Britain to be given a liver transplant. Sadly Ben died just over a year later, in March 1985, aged three and a half.

The most dramatic impact on public awareness came in autumn 1994, following the drive-by shooting in southern Italy of a 7-year-old from California. Nicholas Green's parents – Reginald, a former Fleet Street journalist, and Margaret – agreed to donation and five very sick Italians received new organs and two people were given the boy's corneas. Within a few years of his death, organ donation in Italy had almost tripled, a phenomenon known as the 'Nicholas effect'. Meanwhile, in memory of their son, the Greens set up the Nicholas Green Foundation, published a book and sold thousands of videos – all to promote organ and tissue donation worldwide. 'It never fails to amaze me,' said Reg Green, 'that a small, 7-year-old boy has touched and changed so many lives.'

Here in Britain a system which has developed in a somewhat piecemeal fashion over the past half-century or so is becoming more coherent. However, whether the increase in organ donation predicted by the Organ Donation Taskforce will meet the requirement is by no means certain. Also, it has to be said that a sudden plethora of donated organs could prove embarrassing, because there is still a shortage both of facilities and of suitably experienced medical, nursing and ancillary staff; in particular, some senior transplant surgeons are now approaching retirement. While the Taskforce has signposted the way to major improvements, the need for new donors remains urgent.

June 2011

Chapter 1

The History of Transplantation: Piecemeal Progress

It is no great surprise that organ and tissue transplantation – the transfer of body parts from one person to another – continues to notch up far more media headlines than any other medical enterprise. True, much of the early controversy (remember Christiaan Barnard?) has faded away. Yet the dilemma of donation remains: the fact that one person has to die in order for another to live. Or, increasingly these days, a fit person is whisked into the operating theatre to surrender all or part of an organ to save someone else's life. Also, of course, there are some experimental procedures – face transplants, for instance – which are still fairly controversial.

Spare parts surgery is by no means a recent phenomenon. Mention of skin grafting appears in a Sanskrit text dating back to the second or third century BC. The term 'transplant' is thought to have been introduced by the renowned Scottish surgeon John Hunter (1728–93) in relation to animal experiments. Another Scottish surgeon, William MacEwen of Glasgow, reported the first successful bone graft in 1881. The oldest transplant procedure – and still the most widely practised – is corneal grafting, which was pioneered in the small Moravian town of Olmutz, in what is now the Czech Republic, in 1905. Here an Austrian eye surgeon, Eduard Zirm, took the corneas from an 11-year-old boy whose sight could not be saved to treat Alois Golgar, a labourer who had been blinded in an accident involving caustic lime.

Modern transplantation, of course, developed piecemeal following extensive research and experimentation in the many specialised fields which underpin clinical medicine. In Vienna in 1901, for instance, Karl Landsteiner paved the way to safer blood transfusions with the discovery of the three main blood groups: A, B and O. In the US in the early years of the twentieth century, pioneers included the French surgeon Alexis Carrel and his US associate Charles Guthrie, working at the Rockefeller Institute in New York. Besides switching around dogs' hearts, they developed techniques for reconnecting severed blood vessels (surgical anastomosis), which would be essential to major surgery in general and certainly to transplant operations.

A controversial figure obsessed with eugenics, Carrel received the Nobel Prize for his work in 1912 and two years later he informed the International Surgical Association: 'The surgical side of transplantation of organs is completed as we are now able to perform transplantation of organs with perfect ease ... All our efforts must now be directed toward the biological methods which will prevent the reaction of the organism against foreign tissue.'

However, almost two decades were to pass before anyone tried transplanting organs in human beings. The first to do so was a Russian surgeon, Yu Yu Voronoy, working in the Ukraine. Between 1933 and 1939 he made six attempts to graft cadaver kidneys into very sick patients, all of which failed. Next, in 1946, US surgeons used a cadaver graft in a bid to save a patient who was in acute kidney failure owing to septicaemia. This worked only in that the patient's own kidneys resumed their function within two days.

Throughout these early years the major problem was that of rejection, the body's destructive response to 'foreign' tissue. Although the phenomenon was widely recognised, no one understood how it came about. One of the first people to make sense of it was the late Sir Peter Medawar who, during World War II, probed the failure of skin grafts used in the treatment of severely burned airmen. He observed that rejection arises where donor and recipient do not possess identical genes. It became clear from this seminal work that grafts were being attacked by the immune system which had evolved to protect us from disease.

By the mid-twentieth century the rejection phenomenon was still poorly understood and not yet amenable to manipulation.

Consequently, in 1953, when surgeons in Paris made the first attempt at grafting a kidney from a living donor – mother to son – the organ functioned well for three weeks, until rejection set in.

The world's first successful organ transplant only came about the following year when surgeons at what was then the Peter Bent Brigham Hospital in Boston, Massachusetts, sidestepped the rejection issue altogether by operating on identical twins. They removed one of Ronald Herrick's kidneys and grafted it into his brother, Richard, who was dying of kidney failure. Ronald made an uneventful recovery and lived quite normally with a single kidney for a further forty-seven years; Richard, who married his recovery room nurse, survived for a further eight years before succumbing to heart failure.

This historic operation established the procedure still in use today, whereby in most cases the failed kidneys are left in place and the donor organ is inserted in the recipient's lower abdomen, usually on the right-hand side; it is connected via the ureter to the bladder. Once the blood vessels are connected and circulation is established, the grafted kidney may begin producing urine before the surgeons have had time to close, although some grafts may not function for several weeks.

As paired organs, the kidneys were the natural choice for early experimenters. Surgically, they were always a good bet because of their relatively simple blood supply and the fact that the transplanted kidney often begins to function with gratifying rapidity. Nevertheless, except in the case of identical twins, further attempts at kidney grafting over the next few years ended in failure. The survival rate barely improved even when patients were exposed to total body irradiation (TBI) – first used in Paris in 1958 – to knock out the immune system and anti-cancer drugs to combat rejection. With their natural defences obliterated, most kidney recipients died from infection.

The early 1960s, however, brought a number of advances which would transform kidney grafting from a hazardous, last-chance procedure to a respectable treatment for a wide range of kidney diseases. First came the introduction of tissue typing – matching donor and recipient for compatibility in order to minimise the strength of the immune response. Also, kidney dialysis, developed in occupied Holland during World War II, became available on a routine basis so that patients in renal failure could be supported mechanically and maintained in the best possible condition for transplant surgery.

Then came the major breakthrough which did most to boost graft survival: the appearance of the first effective anti-rejection drug, azathioprine, in 1962. A year later the steroid drug prednisone was brought into use in combination with azathioprine, and this two-drug regimen formed the basis of immunosuppressive therapy for the next two decades. Various other immunosuppressive measures were used in addition, including removal of the spleen, but none yielded any significant further improvement. Finally, in 1980, came an advance which would send the survival rate spiralling. This was the introduction of ciclosporin, a powerful new anti-rejection drug derived from a soil fungus. In fact, the addition of this drug to the immunosuppressive armoury would soon enhance survival in all transplant categories.

The latest development on the renal front, taking transplantation into the precision age, came in 2008, when US surgeons staged the world's first robot-assisted kidney transplant. The patient, who had suffered renal failure as a complication of Type 1 diabetes, received a kidney donated by her husband, who, coincidentally, happened to be a good match. A statement from the St Barnabas Medical Center in Livingston, New Jersey, said that, utilising the latest robotic system, 'a laparoscopic camera and robotic probes are inserted into the patient through several small incisions. Pencil-sized probes translate the surgeon's hand movements and adjust themselves to compensate for the natural tremor of the human hand. For the patient, robot-assisted surgery is safe, minimally invasive and offers faster recovery time.'

The largest incision through which the donor kidney is inserted is, at 5 cm (2 in), only about a third the length of a conventional 'open' kidney transplant incision. The clinical team, who have since done more of these keyhole procedures, insist that robot technology is a remarkable surgical tool. Above all, it is associated with a lower incidence of the most frequent post-operative complications – wound infection and bleeding.

Meanwhile, back in the dark days of the 1960s, the results of pancreas transplant remained dismal. The initial attempt, at the University of Minnesota in 1966, and a further thirteen at the same centre over the next four years, all proved disappointing, with only one graft functioning for more than a year. Here again survival really only began to pick up with the arrival of ciclosporin.

Pancreas transplantation was developed to relieve severe diabetes. The idea is to free the recipient with Type 1 (early onset) diabetes from dependence on insulin and also to limit the secondary complications associated with the disease, which include blindness, kidney disease and heart trouble. There is the temptation to replace the pancreas well before the kidneys fail, but doctors have to bear in mind that diabetes is not immediately life-threatening. Therefore, the benefits of pancreatic transplantation have to be weighed against the risks of surgery and a lifetime of immunosuppressive drugs.

In the UK, where the first pancreas transplant was carried out in Cambridge in 1979, enthusiasm for the procedure only began to pick up from about the mid-1980s. The pancreas is sometimes transplanted on its own in diabetic patients who are experiencing frequent and severe 'hypos', with the risk of coma and death. More common, however, is simultaneous pancreas-kidney transplant (SPK), the procedure performed for patients with Type 1 diabetes who are also in kidney failure. For SPK, first-year survival is about 85 per cent.

A tantalising alternative sometimes tried for patients with unstable Type 1 diabetes is islet transplantation. In this much simpler procedure, insulin-producing islet cells of the pancreas are injected through the abdominal wall into the portal vein, a vessel which carries nutrient-rich blood from the intestine to the liver. Researchers began working on this in the 1960s but first attempts, in the 1990s, had a very low success rate. However, in 1999, a team at the University of Alberta in Edmonton ran a clinical trial using enhanced techniques to collect and prepare the islet cells; it also featured an improved anti-rejection regimen. This trial proved 100 per cent successful and since then the Edmonton protocol has been taken up, and in some cases adapted, at centres around the world.

Patients receiving an islet cell transplant can either reduce their insulin or stop using it altogether. The trouble is that these very fragile cells account for only about 2 to 3 per cent of pancreatic tissue and so harvesting specific cells in sufficient quantity is difficult. In the UK two specialist laboratories have been set up to isolate cells from cadaver donors and prepare them for transplantation.

A variation on this theme is occasionally used as a last resort for patients suffering the excruciating pain of pancreatitis, inflammation of the pancreas. If the pancreas is removed, the patient is rendered diabetic. However, a recent option is for the pancreas to be removed and the healthy islet cells salvaged so that they can be injected into the patient's portal vein. Here again there is the problem of finding sufficient cells, particularly from a pancreas which is already damaged, and patients mostly remain insulin-dependent.

Transplantation of the largest and most versatile of internal organs, the liver, got off to an even worse start than renal transplantation had done a decade earlier. Following experimental work in animals in the 1950s, this formidable procedure was first undertaken in a human being in Denver, Colorado, in 1963. The patient, a 3-year-old boy with biliary atresia, died on the operating table. Further attempts were made at centres in the US and France, but it was not until 1967 that, also in Denver, the first successful outcome was reported. Britain's first liver transplant took place a year later.

For more than a decade the best one-year survival rate reported for liver grafting was only 50 per cent. For the most part the operation remained frankly heroic, something of a last-ditch measure to be performed only on patients who were already on the brink of death. It is no wonder that so many of these early recipients died, for at this stage the operation was truly forbidding, often involving the replacement of many pints of blood. A major problem was that, since organs could not yet be taken from ventilated donors, many of the organs acquired for grafting were in poor condition. Consequently, any patient undergoing what was still a highly experimental procedure had to run the gauntlet of technical complications, rejection or infection, all of which could lead to loss of the graft. This meant either a re-transplant – at one point some centres were performing these at a rate of almost 20 per cent – or death of the patient.

Gradually, the technical problems associated with the surgery itself and with the post-operative care of recipients were overcome and, of course, by the mid-1970s brainstem death protocols (see Chapter 2) had been introduced, enabling the retrieval of organs from ventilated patients. This automatically increased the number and viability of donor livers becoming available for transplant. The trouble was that, because of the need to use donated organs within a few hours, liver transplants were being performed against a backdrop of flashing lights, with surgical teams rushing between donor and recipient hospitals and often operating through the night.

Even if they survived the operation, desperately ill recipients were in poor shape to withstand the high doses of steroids being given to suppress the immune system and so prevent rejection. By 1980, the average one-year survival after liver transplantation was still only 30 per cent. Here again, use of ciclosporin brought phenomenal improvements in survival, just as it had for other transplants.

An effect of all this was that transplant centres could open their doors to a much wider selection of liver patients rather than the spectral, often comatose figures who had peopled the earlier scenario. Those with progressive disease could now be taken onto the waiting list, and hopefully transplanted, before becoming so debilitated that it would be touch and go whether they would make it through surgery; so could patients in acute liver failure – previously also considered a poor surgical risk. Now, too, liver transplantation could be recommended for categories previously excluded: the very young (below 10 kg in body weight) and the elderly.

Finally, an important logistical breakthrough was the introduction in the late 1980s of a perfusion fluid, developed at the University of Wisconsin, which could extend the time that donated livers could be stored without risk of deterioration. The availability of the UW solution, as it became known, meant that surgical teams no longer needed to tackle transplantation at breakneck speed. Today, with almost 700 people in the UK undergoing liver transplantation each year, the one-year survival rate is 90 per cent; higher still in children.

For some years surgeons have been performing split-liver grafts – 'cut-downs' – from adult livers. This has proved a life-saver for babies in particular, since so few donor livers of appropriate size become available for them. The segment fulfils the functions of a normal baby liver and grows with its new owner. The use of split livers, of course, eases the supply situation by enabling more than one transplant from a single cadaver donation.

A recent alternative, mainly for patients in acute liver failure, is auxiliary liver grafting, where a portion of donor liver is inserted alongside the patient's own liver. This enables the native liver to rest and recuperate over time and saves the patient having to spend the rest of his or her life on anti-rejection drugs.

Meanwhile, there have been some promising results from the use of stem-cell therapy to treat liver disease. Stem cells, which can be obtained from blood or bone marrow, have the potential to turn into many different types of body tissue. Experimental work has shown that, introduced into a diseased liver, the cells somehow promote its regeneration.

As with kidneys and livers, the early days of heart transplantation, too, were conspicuously disastrous. In 1964, a team at the University of Mississippi was poised to attempt the first human heart transplant into a 64-year-old diabetic patient who was close to death from advanced heart disease. When no donor heart could be found, the surgeon used the heart from a laboratory chimpanzee instead. The heart beat independently for ninety minutes but proved too small to support the demands of a human patient.

This exercise attracted widespread disapproval, but even so several further attempted xenografts – transplanting animal organs into humans – were made using hearts taken from sheep, baboons and chimpanzees. None of these adult recipients lived for more than a few days. Possibly most notorious was the Baby Fae case in 1984, when a baby girl was given a baboon heart at Loma Linda University Medical Center in California. The child survived for twenty days.

Then, in 1967, leading researchers in the field, who had been experimenting with cardiac transplantation for years at Stanford University in California, were pipped at the post when the South African surgeon Christiaan Barnard performed the world's first human heart transplant using a human donor. The patient, 54-year-old Louis Washkansky, seemed to spend most of the remaining eighteen days of his life in front of television cameras before finally dying from pneumonia.

Not the least controversial aspect of all this was the fact that Barnard himself had certified the death of the donor, a road accident victim. In these early days the names of organ donors were often released and it became known that Washkansky had received the heart of a white South African woman called Denise Darvall (one of whose kidneys was transplanted into a 10-year-old coloured boy). Nevertheless, the operation generated a global fanfare of publicity and the South African surgeon became a celebrity overnight.

Rather less attention was paid to another operation carried out on the same day: the use of the heart from a 19-month-old anencephalic infant – born with the upper part of the brain missing – for a transplant at Maimonides Medical Center in Brooklyn, US. The result was said to have been an 'unequivocal failure'.

Further attempts at cardiac transplantation were made in no less than seventeen countries. Britain's first heart transplant took place at what was the National Heart Hospital (now the Royal Brompton National Heart and Lung Hospital) in London in May 1968. Here, concern was such that the senior anaesthetist spent the first post-operative night on a trolley beside the patient. The recipient in this case – only the tenth heart transplant in the world – was kept in theatre for a fortnight for close monitoring. He survived for forty-five days.

As one of the surgical team told a Wellcome Trust meeting almost three decades later: 'The thing that strikes me now, looking back on it, was the relative freedom that everybody had to do it. If one was making a world-shaking advance now, one would probably have to apply to statutory bodies for permission, acquire the funds and get it approved by many committees.'

In general, however, the results of cardiac transplantation in those days were catastrophic, largely owing to a failure in the assessment and treatment of rejection. Internationally, most centres imposed a moratorium on further attempts, but the Stanford University team, led by the late Norman Shumway, persisted and were able to demonstrate that, with skilled post-operative management, transplantation could be a viable answer for the failing heart. With hearts, as with livers and kidneys, dramatic improvements in survival would only come with the introduction of ciclosporin. Heart transplantation recommenced in Britain in the late 1970s.

Heart transplantation is offered mainly for coronary heart disease (CHD) or cardiomyopathy, which is a failure of the heart muscle, in some cases owing to a viral infection. Cardiomyopathy tends to strike a younger population of patients than CHD and often results in much more rapid deterioration. A 12-year-old girl from South Wales with this condition made history in 2006 by having her heart transplant reversed. A decade earlier she had been facing death from heart failure. This was before a reliable device became available to assist the failing heart. So, in a desperate bid to save her, surgeons grafted a heart from a 5-month-old donor into her chest. This 'piggyback' heart served well until rejection set in late in 2005. It was removed once it was established that the child's own heart had recovered.

The earliest known experiments in cardiopulmonary (heart-lung) transplantation were carried out in dogs in the 1940s by a young Russian surgeon, Vladimir Demikhov, working in Moscow. Most of these animals died because, as it was later discovered, their lungs would not function properly without a nerve supply. However, in human beings and other primates respiratory control is possible even when the nerve supply has been severed. The first successful heart-lung transplant took place at Stanford in 1981. The recipient, a 45-year-old woman, lived for a further five years.

The combined procedure – grafting what is known as a heart-lung block, comprising the heart and both lungs – quickly gained acceptance as a treatment for a number of lung diseases. For several years it was preferred to single or double-lung grafting because heart-lung blocks were easy to 'harvest', the surgery was technically straightforward and there was better healing of the join between the donor and recipient segments of windpipe. However, various centres tried to refine the lung procedure (first attempted back in 1963), not least because it was clearly wasteful to transplant three donor organs into patients who only required one serviceable lung. Some heart-lung recipients, of course – for instance, those with cystic fibrosis – had sound hearts and so these could be removed and transplanted into recipients with heart disease in what became known as the domino procedure.

The first human lung transplant was carried out in Jackson, Mississippi, in 1963. The recipient, a patient with terminal lung cancer who was under sentence of death for murder, died of kidney failure on the eighteenth post-operative day. From then until 1980, more than forty further lung transplants were attempted, in twenty-six centres worldwide, with no real success. Most were 'rescue' attempts on patients who had become ventilator-dependent. Only two lung recipients survived more than a month. Here again, as with heart transplants, a moratorium ensued until ciclosporin became available. Finally, the first successful single lung transplant was carried out at the University of Toronto in 1983.

By the late 1980s, demand for donated hearts had increased and fewer heart-lung blocks were becoming available. By this time, however, techniques of lung grafting had improved considerably and interest in these approaches began to increase. The technique of en bloc double-lung transplantation, pioneered in the mid-1980s, was associated with such complications that it proved to be safer to offer two separate lung transplants, in what became known as bilateral single lung replacement, for patients requiring replacement of both lungs. This is now the commonest lung transplant procedure, performed mostly for cystic fibrosis. Replacement of a single lung is only appropriate where there is no infection.

Today the heart-lung procedure, which was pioneered at Stanford in 1981, is recommended only for the congenital hole-in-the-heart condition known as Eisenmenger's syndrome and for patients with end-stage lung disease with heart involvement. Only five heart-lung transplants were carried out in the UK in the year ending March 2010.

There remains concern that brainstem death, the condition that yields almost all lungs used for grafting, somehow results in damage to the lungs, heightening the risk of rejection in the recipient, and researchers are looking at ways of treating the lungs of potential multi-organ donors to prevent damage. There have been some examples of lungs being used from patients whose hearts have stopped in accident and emergency departments (see Chapter 3). However, for logistical reasons this is not always an option.

With the exception of kidneys, none of these major procedures would be possible without the life-support technology that has evolved over the past sixty-odd years. Positive-pressure ventilators, for instance, used in intensive care units for short-term maintenance of brainstem-dead donors, provide a means of keeping organs perfused with oxygenated blood and, therefore, viable for transplantation; the ventilator is used, too, to sustain the recipient's breathing during and for a while after transplant surgery. In addition, the heart-lung machine, introduced in 1953, is essential in major procedures to keep a blood supply going while the recipient's own circulation is interrupted. Various devices may be used, in addition to drugs, to assist the failing heart in the run-up to transplantation.

The small bowel was one of the last major organs to be transplanted successfully. This is the largest segment of the digestive system, growing up to six and a half metres (22 ft) in the adult. The operation is a difficult one, developed for patients suffering from irreversible failure of the small intestine, including short-gut (or short-bowel) syndrome where, owing to injury or disease, there is too little functional intestine to meet the body's nutritional needs. Unable to absorb nutrients in the usual way, these patients are dependent on artificial feeding (parenteral nutrition), receiving food in liquid form by way of a catheter inserted into a large vein. Those who cannot eat normally at all are dependent on total parenteral nutrition (TPN). However, there are a number of complications associated with long-term artificial feeding, including metabolic problems and recurrent infection. Also, a significant proportion of patients (children especially) die from TPN-related liver failure.

It is for this reason that workers at the University of Minnesota began to experiment with small bowel grafting in the late 1950s. The first attempts to transplant the small bowel in human beings were made in the mid-1960s but, as with other pioneer transplants, the outcomes were universally grim. In the days before there were safe and effective techniques for parenteral feeding, surgeons had to operate on very frail, undernourished patients. Also, intestinal grafts are more susceptible to rejection and infection than other organ transplants and so many recipients died of sepsis.

The operation was abandoned for some years and only revived following the introduction of ciclosporin. The first prolonged survival – from a combined liver-small bowel transplant – was reported from the University of Western Ontario in 1988. Survival rates were slow to improve, but picked up measurably from 1992 with the arrival of a newer immunosuppressive drug, tacrolimus, which is more effective than ciclosporin in small bowel recipients. Currently, survival figures are approaching those seen with lung and liver transplantation and this infrequently used procedure is seen as an increasingly acceptable option for patients suffering the long-term complications of TPN.

The small bowel may be grafted in isolation or, where there is extensive abdominal disease, as part of what is known as a multi-visceral or radical 'cluster' transplant involving other organs, such as the liver, pancreas, stomach and colon. Often controversial, these complex procedures, in which multiple organs may be transplanted en bloc or individually, were developed mainly in the US from the mid-1960s onwards.

In Britain there was pressure to develop a multi-visceral programme when, in June 1992, a toddler from Manchester had to be flown to Pittsburgh for life-saving surgery. Laura Davies was born with a congenital defect (gastroschisis), where part of the bowel protrudes through the abdominal wall. She was unable to digest food normally and her liver was also affected. An appeal raised more than £750,000 for the trip (including a generous contribution from King Fahd of Saudi Arabia) and Laura underwent a lengthy operation to graft a new liver and small bowel.

Back at home, Laura's jaundice disappeared and she seemed to make a good recovery. But then cancerous growths began to appear on the internal organs – a side-effect of the very high doses of drugs she had been given to combat rejection. The small bowel showed signs of failing and her body began to reject the donated organs. A year after surgery Laura was flown back to Pittsburgh. Surgeons then decided on a cluster of six organs – liver, pancreas, stomach, small and large bowel and both kidneys – in what would be the most ambitious multiple transplant ever attempted.

Again, the 5-year-old made a good recovery and returned home. However, the cancer soon returned and Laura's death in November 1993 (six weeks after surgery) prompted a torrent of criticism. Even the surgeon who had led the Pittsburgh team conceded that she may have been exposed to too much suffering. But the episode also triggered moves to begin to provide a small bowel programme in the UK. The first small bowel transplant in a child in Europe was carried out at the Birmingham Children's Hospital in 1993.

Arguably the world's most prolific transplant hospital is Jackson Memorial Medical Center in Miami, which has a long record of cluster procedures. One of the most ambitious, performed in 1997, was a seven-transplant endeavour to save an Italian infant. This little girl was still alive – and apparently doing well – in January 2004, when surgeons at Jackson Memorial broke their own cluster record by performing a twelve-hour marathon to transplant no less than eight organs. Also from Genoa, also suffering a potentially fatal disorder of the digestive system, was 6-month-old Alessia di Matteo, who received a liver, small and large intestine, pancreas, stomach, spleen and two kidneys; a further kidney transplant was undertaken in April. However, this second infant died in January the following year.

No less controversial are some of the newer experimental procedures attempted over the last decade or so. These are reconstructive exercises, using cadaver tissues to replace or rebuild parts of the body which are missing or damaged. Critics make the point that these operations are not life-saving. They expose otherwise healthy people to all the risks of transplantation generally, including lifelong immunosuppression, the possibility of developing drug-associated cancer and the constant fear of rejection.

The most emotive of the new procedures is transplantation of the face for people who have been left grossly disfigured by accident or disease. Traditionally, such patients have had to undergo countless operations to try to make good the damage. Sometimes, reattachment surgery is possible. The most famous case of this kind was that of a 9-year-old Indian girl whose face and scalp were ripped off in a threshing machine accident in 1994. Sandeep Kaur's family had the presence of mind to put the damaged tissue into a plastic bag and take it and the child to hospital – a three-and-a-half-hour journey by moped – where it was successfully reattached.

Since then a number of centres have experimented with face transplants on cadavers donated for medical research in order to answer the key question: whether or not the grafted recipient takes on the appearance of the donor. This does not happen because, of course, the two individuals would have totally different bone structure and musculature. Even so, initially there was reluctance to replace the face of a living patient, not least because of the fear that the introduction of face transplants would be counterproductive, deterring some people from agreeing to donate any tissue at all.

Finally, French surgeons took the initiative by performing the world's first face transplant at a hospital in Amiens in November 2005. The recipient was 38-year-old Isabelle Dinoire, whose face apparently had been eaten away by her dog while she was lying in a coma. The transplant in this case was a partial one: a triangular graft, which included the nose, lips and chin, was lifted from a brain-dead woman who was lying in a hospital in Lille, still on a ventilator. Besides skin and fat, the graft also comprised nerves, muscle and blood vessels. A flap of skin was also taken from one of the donor's forearms, to be positioned onto Isabelle's chest as a 'sentinel graft', from which biopsies could be taken when necessary so as to limit damage to her new face.

Besieged by the world's media, Isabelle then suffered two brief bouts of rejection, on the eighteenth post-operative day and again at about seven months, and she also had to be treated for kidney failure owing to the powerful immunosuppressants she had been prescribed. The

French medical team, reporting on the outcome at eighteen months post-surgery, described the 'functional and aesthetic' results of the transplant as 'satisfactory'.

Further face transplants have followed in France, the US and China, and it is partly their success which prompted a change of heart at the Royal College of Surgeons (RCS), which had vetoed the whole idea in 2003. A second report (2006) from the RCS working party gave cautious approval to a start-up programme in Britain, while warning that the procedure was still experimental. 'We are anxious to avoid a repetition of the media and medical frenzy that accompanied the first heart transplants in the late 1960s,' cautioned the RCS.

There was quite a media circus surrounding the first ever successful hand transplant, carried out in France in 1998 by the same surgeon who would later give Isabelle Dinoire her new face. New Zealander Clint Hallam received a hand from a young motorcyclist who had died in an accident. The hand and its new owner pursued a chequered course and at length Hallam asked for the hand to be removed.

Face, hand and various other transplants which feature more than one tissue – skin, fat, muscle, nerves, blood vessels – are known as composite tissue allografts (CTAs). They rely on microsurgical skills, developed in the 1970s, which enable the exquisitely fine work needed to connect nerves and minute blood vessels. But the team at London's Royal Free Hospital, who are poised to initiate the UK's face transplant programme, has warned that there is approximately a 5 per cent failure rate whenever minute blood vessels are grafted microscopically. This means that, irrespective of immunosuppression, the likelihood of failure is of the order of 5 per cent.

One of the major obstacles to CTA procedures, as the Royal College of Surgeons report points out, is the vulnerability of the skin to rejection. Skin, after all, is the body's protective barrier and as such it is immunologically highly active. Chronic rejection has occurred in a number of hand transplants and is seen in up to 50 per cent of organ transplants within five years. The Royal College predicts that it could develop in 30 to 50 per cent of face transplants. At worst, the recipient developing chronic rejection ultimately would have to endure repeated skin grafts or a re-transplant.

A possible breakthrough which bypasses the rejection issue altogether came with a new kind of graft used to treat a 30-year-old woman with a diseased airway. This procedure – the first ever bio-engineered human transplant – was developed by scientists from Bristol, Milan and Padua. A 7 cm (2.75 in) length of trachea, taken from a woman who had died of a brain haemorrhage, was stripped of all the donor cells, leaving only a cartilage scaffold. This was then re-seeded with tissue grown from the recipient's own bone marrow stem cells.

Claudia Costello's left main bronchus had collapsed owing to tuberculosis. Breathless even at rest, she agreed to the experimental graft – in preference to losing the lung – and was transplanted at the Hospital Clinic in Barcelona in June 2008. Within a month of surgery, the new airway had developed its own blood supply and the Spanish medical team said that, with no sign of rejection, Claudia was once more able to lead a normal life, free of the need to take anti-rejection medication.

Specialists in the field have welcomed the new technique and believe it could be applied to other procedures, such as laryngeal (voice box) transplant. There have only been two laryngeal transplants to date, in the US in 1998 and again in early 2011, and now a pan-European team is researching the possibility of developing a new bioengineering procedure for the many people – about 1,000 a year in Britain alone – whose voice boxes are lost to injury or disease.

Predictably there has been lively media interest, too, in the limited attempts to transplant various reproductive organs, including the ovaries, womb and penis. The first successful ovary transplant, carried out in St Louis, Missouri, in 2007, was one between identical twins. The recipient twin, who previously had been infertile for twelve years, was able to conceive and give birth to a daughter in London the following year.

The first attempt to transplant the womb took place in Saudi Arabia (where surrogacy is illegal) in 2000. However, the graft had to be removed after three months owing to the formation of a blood clot. The idea with womb transplants is for the donated organ to be removed and discarded once the recipient has borne children so that immunosuppression is no longer necessary.

The world's first and only penis transplant took place at the Guangzhou General Hospital in China in 2005. The 44-year-old recipient, having lost his own member in an accident, received the penis of man half his age who had been declared brainstem-dead. However, the surgeon reported that the donor organ, though healthy, had to be removed on the fifteenth post-operative day because of a 'severe psychological problem' which had arisen for the donor and his wife.

Certainly transplantation is one of the greatest medical success stories of our time. Little more than half a century after the first successful kidney transplant, surgeons can transplant almost any type of body tissue from tiny chips of bone to the great organs of the chest and abdomen. The solid organ transplants have emerged from the experimental category to become routine procedures, 'treatments of choice'. With all this high-profile activity, though, too often overlooked are the more humdrum grafts – of tissues such as skin, bone, joints, nerves and corneas – which can restore mobility, sensation or sight or prevent the loss of a limb. Other than blood, bone is now the most frequently grafted tissue worldwide.

Chapter 2

A State Beyond Coma

The heartbeating donor, someone who is brainstem-dead but whose circulation is kept going artificially in intensive care, has been the primary source of organs for transplant for more than three decades. The first formal description of brainstem death appeared in a medical journal in 1959. In what one eminent British neurologist described as 'a masterpiece of clinical observation', two French specialists, Pierre Mollaret and Marcel Goulon, identified what they termed *coma dépassé* – a state 'beyond coma'. The detail they gave immediately rang bells with doctors in every country with advanced medical facilities. For, with new methods of resuscitation and life support, they, too, had been witnessing the apparent survival of an increasing number of deeply comatose patients – victims of brain injury or illness – who could no longer breathe on their own account.

What all these doctors had been seeing was the death of the most primitive part of the brain, the brainstem, which controls basic life processes such as breathing and circulation. This is something which occurs when the brainstem is deprived of its blood supply (and, therefore, of oxygen) or when other parts of the brain are damaged by disease or injury. Whatever the cause, the effect is swelling of the brain. The trouble is that, housed within the bony confines of the skull, the brain has little room to expand. If the swelling does not respond to treatment, pressure builds up inside the skull and brain tissue is forced down through the small opening in the base of the skull where it meets the spinal cord. This compresses the brainstem, shutting off its blood supply. If the pressure continues, the brainstem dies.

In the past, patients with overwhelming damage in this vital area would simply have stopped breathing and that would have been the end. But by the 1950s they could be put promptly on mechanical ventilators before a shortage of oxygen caused the heart to stop. Transferred to the new intensive care units (ICUs) being pioneered at this time, these 'living cadavers' (as they were originally known in the States) appeared as if in sleep. Pink and warm to the touch, they were sometimes seen to make sudden movements – raising one or both arms off the bed, occasionally turning the head from side to side – and onlookers were reassured by the rhythmic rise and fall of the chest wall. Yet, even with meticulous care, these patients all suffered the same fate: within a few days their hearts stopped beating.

Today, of course, it is recognised that such patients had in fact been dead ever since they lost the capacity to breathe. A Home Counties GP who lost his medical student son in this way following a road accident explains: 'When the brainstem is damaged beyond repair, the delicate chemical balance of the body (on which all life depends) begins to go out of control. This is one of the reasons why "drips" are used in life support. The fluids partly correct the chemical imbalances which are occurring. However, eventually the chemistry of a body with a dead brainstem goes completely out of control and all the processes of life, including the heartbeat, stop within about a week.'

To this extent, brainstem death is a stark reminder of the fact that, in most cases, death is a process, not an event. As Lewis Thomas pointed out in his book *Lives of a Cell* (Bantam, 1974): 'Death is not a sudden, all-at-once affair; cells go down in sequence, one by one.'

So here, at the dawn of life-support technology, the dying process was being extended artificially; in this context, all that ICUs were doing was ventilating cadavers. Nevertheless, for years many units continued to support comatose, apnoeic patients (those unable to breathe on their own) until their hearts stopped. As time went by this was done less in the hope that they might recover than because doctors lacked the scientific data needed to justify withdrawal of treatment. The first person to exploit this novel source of organs for transplantation, in June 1963, was a Belgian surgeon, Guy Alexandre, working at the St Pierre Hospital in Louvain. In what was seen at the time as a highly controversial initiative, he removed a kidney from a brainstem-dead donor for grafting.

Elsewhere, it was to be some years before hospital practice gradually began to change – in the light of mounting evidence from many countries that destruction of the brainstem is indeed irreversible. In the US, the first formal affirmation that irreversible damage to the brainstem results in death was issued by the Harvard Medical Committee in 1968. Finally, in the mid-1970s, British neurologists, anaesthetists and other medical specialists led the world in actually defining brainstem death in order to be able to discontinue futile treatment. Their criteria incorporated simple tests (see Appendix I) which could be carried out at the bedside.

The tests explore the viability of the brainstem in two ways. In the first place, they establish whether or not certain nerve reflexes are working, for as one of the specialists who led their development has pointed out, testing these reflexes 'probes the brainstem slice by slice, as if it were salami'. In addition, they determine whether or not the patient can breathe unaided.

Of course, not all ventilated patients in deep coma are candidates for testing. Some do not meet the preconditions laid down in the UK code of practice because their situation is associated with a cause which is potentially reversible. This includes patients in coma owing to the prolonged effects of certain drugs, hypothermia or some gross disturbance of body chemistry. Cases which meet the preconditions are those arising from a known cause of irreversible damage, including: head injury, brain haemorrhage, brain tumour or failure of the oxygen supply to the brain as, for example, in cardiac arrest or suffocation.

Once an unconscious, ventilated patient is admitted to the intensive care unit, the length of time he or she remains on life support will depend on the history and the results of scans and other tests. Normally, medical staff would not consider brainstem death as a possible diagnosis until at least six hours had elapsed; often the interval is much longer. When the coma persists, and the clinical picture suggests a brainstem catastrophe, the code calls for testing to be undertaken by two experienced doctors, at least one of whom must be a consultant and neither of whom are involved in transplantation.

Some other countries, including the US, use the term 'brain-death' as opposed to 'brainstem death'. They go to considerable lengths to demonstrate death of the brain as a whole, using a battery of tests and scans which are not required in this country. The UK protocol was built on the elegantly simple observation that death of the brainstem is by implication death of the brain as a whole. Interestingly, wide variation in practice has been shown in the US, where the Uniform Determination of Death Act of 1981 (US) did not lay down guidelines for the determination of brain-death. A study outlined at an American Academy of Neurology (AAN) meeting in October 2007 reported a 'huge mismatch' between AAN guidelines and the parameters in use at individual hospitals.

Some people have difficulty grasping the distinction between brainstem death and some other states of unresponsiveness. It is sometimes confused, for instance, with the vegetative state, where the victim may never regain awareness. In the vegetative state it is most or all of the cortex – the brain's 'grey matter' – which is destroyed, while the sturdier cells of the brainstem continue to maintain vital processes. The vegetative patient, therefore, breathes spontaneously and may survive indefinitely; the brainstem-dead patient has lost the capacity to breathe.

Clearly, the concept of brainstem death and the protocols surrounding its diagnosis were not dreamed up to advance transplantation. They were developed to resolve an appalling dilemma which had been thrown up by the introduction of advanced medical technology. If, suddenly, all transplant activity were to cease, doctors would still need to diagnose brainstem death. However, the arrival of the heartbeating donor provided transplant surgeons with an ideal source of organs. Hospital shorthand for donation in these circumstances is DBD (donation after brainstem death).

For relatives and friends, summoned perhaps to some distant hospital, seeing a loved one in this macabre condition is frankly a nightmare. What is so bewildering is the suddenness of it all (and sometimes the violence) and always the unreality, for the patient looks so alive. Many people have great difficulty reconciling what they see – a body which is pink and warm and apparently breathing – with what they are being told. Before coming to accept the finality of the diagnosis, they may question repeatedly how their loved ones can be dead when they are still breathing, whether or not they feel any pain, whether recovery would be possible if they were left on the ventilator indefinitely ...

In fact, over the years the phenomenon of 'chronic brain-death' – where a minority of brainstem-dead patients have been found to 'survive' far longer than the norm – has been seen from time to time. In 1998, a researcher in California reported a meta-analysis of 175 cases of patients whose hearts had continued to beat for at least a week. In 80 of these artificially maintained patients, the heartbeat was preserved for at least two weeks; in approximately 44 for four weeks; in 20 for two months; and in 7 for an astounding six months. The author found that adults in this series had all arrested within four months, whereas in children the heart seemed capable of beating almost indefinitely.

There have been a few notable instances of pregnant women diagnosed brainstem-dead who have been maintained long enough for the fetus to mature sufficiently to be viable. The longest reported case, from Burlington, Vermont, is that of a 30-year-old woman fatally injured in a road accident in 1989. She was diagnosed brainstem-dead at 15 weeks' gestation but maintained in intensive care for 107 days until a healthy baby boy, weighing 1.55 kg (3.5 lb), could be delivered by Caesarean section at 32 weeks; subsequently, he was seen to be developing normally. The first UK case of this kind was reported from Middlesbrough three years earlier.

By far the longest known chronic brain-death survival is that of a 4-year-old in Nebraska who, in the days before a vaccine became available, developed meningitis. Comatose on admission to hospital, he was pronounced brain-dead. There was absolutely no doubt about this: his brain had swollen to such an extent that the skull sutures (joints where the bony plates meet) had split. However, the family would not agree to removal of life support and so the child was kept going for the next two decades, cared for at various times in hospital, in a chronic care facility for ventilator-dependent patients and at home. After his final period of hospitalisation, his mother decided against any further attempts at resuscitation and his heart eventually stopped in January 2004.

Chronic brain-death is exceedingly rare and there is no question of any residual brain activity in any of these victims. In the Nebraska case the post-mortem findings confirmed the fact that the meningitis twenty years earlier had caused the child's death. The brain was seen to be mostly calcified, its structures barely recognisable. In any such case, of course, if the ventilator were to be disconnected the patient's heart would stop within a few minutes.

Intensive care staff normally identify a potential donor some time before the question of donation is broached with the relatives. At this point it is usual to notify the specialist nurses in organ donation (SNODs, formerly known as donor transplant co-ordinators), key figures in the unfolding process who handle the complex logistics of donation as well as helping to care for the bereaved family and to support ICU staff. Already the family will have been told the outlook is poor and it is at this point that a doctor (usually a consultant) explains the need to carry out brainstem death tests. The tests, performed by two doctors and lasting at most half an hour, will demonstrate whether or not there is any life remaining in the brainstem.

There are mixed views on the question of relatives witnessing the tests. Some doctors in charge of ICUs (in the UK, mainly anaesthetists) are in favour; some are not. A survey of twenty-eight neurotrauma ICUs in the UK, reported in the year 2000, found that 32 per cent of consultants and 42 per cent of nurses had experience of family members being present during the tests. Of these medical and nursing staff, 69 per cent felt the experience had helped the relatives.

Researchers from an ICU at one of the northern hospitals five years later interviewed twenty-seven adults who had witnessed the tests. It was a year after bereavement and, of these, eighteen said that they knew beforehand that death had occurred; the remaining nine still had some hope that the tests would reveal a possibility of the patient's survival; three people were still 'confused' about the implications of the test findings. Naturally, not all relatives want to see the tests being performed, but it is interesting that some people who did not witness them developed fantasies about what might be going on which may have been more disturbing than if they had been present at the bedside.

Of course, there are some people who, despite all the appearances, seem to know instinctively that their relative is dead. A lady from Peterborough recalls the November Saturday night when her eldest daughter was rushed to hospital with multiple injuries from a car accident. The 13 year old was conscious and able to speak on admission, but she deteriorated over the weekend and died, her mother believes, in the early hours of Monday morning. 'I knew exactly the moment she went. I said as much to the nurse, but she seemed a bit taken aback – too upset perhaps to respond.'

In the long hours that followed, awaiting the two series of tests for brainstem death, this lady received immense kindness from the intensive care staff. 'Nothing was too much trouble for them. They were happy to answer all my questions and to explain anything I wanted to know. One of the most wonderful things was that they let me wash my daughter's hair. She had lovely hair, but here it was all matted and dirty from the accident. It meant a lot to me to be able to do that for her.'

When the tests confirm that the brainstem is dead, a second set – identical to the first – is performed as an additional safeguard for the patient (although it has to be said that in the UK there has been no documented case where the findings of the second set overturned those of the first). It is during the interval between the two sets of tests that the question of donation is raised with the family. At first, hospital staff are keen to establish whether or not the patient carries a donor card, has signed up to the NHS Organ Donor Register (see page 137) or has expressed any views on organ donation. Sometimes this is known; sometimes not.

However, they are also keen to know the wishes of family members, especially, of course, the next of kin. Also, if the patient has lived closely with someone unrelated, the views of this person, too, are sought. If he or she carried a donor card or signed up to the donor register, no one has the right to overrule those wishes, according to the Human Tissue Act 2004. In practice the family, when available, are always consulted. ICU staff are not immune to the horror of sudden loss and their concern is to ensure that the shock and anguish experienced by family and friends are not compounded in any way.

The Act stipulates that, if the dead person's wishes are not known but he or she has nominated a representative to act for them after death, this person can give consent for donation. If there is no nominated representative, consent can be given by anyone who has been in a 'qualifying relationship' with the dead person immediately before his or her death. The Act ranks such relationships in the following order: spouse or partner (including civil partner); parent or child; brother or sister; grandparent or grandchild; niece or nephew; stepfather or stepmother; half-brother or sister; or friend of long standing.

Within reason there is no pressure of time on people when coming to a decision about organ donation. They are free to raise any questions which may be bothering them, especially perhaps in relation to brainstem death itself – a difficult concept which takes some time to digest. Perhaps the most telling point that intensive care staff can impart is that no patient tested in accordance with the UK code of practice has ever been known to recover. Relatives and friends should be clear in their minds that, irrespective of the donation issue, death will be certified after the first set of brainstem death tests, the formal point of death.

Once the second set is completed, if there is to be no donation, the ventilator will be disconnected and the dead person's heart will stop within a few minutes. Or, if there is consent for donation, one of the SNODs makes arrangements for the retrieval operation, which is invariably carried out in the hospital where the donor is lying. The family may choose to remain at the bedside or, if there is to be a long wait before surgery, they may prefer to go home, possibly returning to the hospital later on to view the body at rest. The ICU nurse remains at the bedside.

In the interval before surgery – usually a maximum of twelve hours – medical and nursing care of the donor is every bit as meticulous as it was in life. Now there is no question of treatment. Instead, the concern is to maintain the organs in as healthy a condition as possible. To do this, ICU staff must ensure that the donor remains adequately oxygenated, minimise loss of body heat, carry out routine hygienic measures, prevent infection and correct any fluid or chemical imbalance which may arise.

At length, all the medical records, including documentation of brainstem death and signed permission for organ donation, are taken with the donor to the operating theatre. Sometimes, a relative who has remained at the bedside may accompany the deceased, taking his or her leave at the entrance to the theatre suite.

The retrieval operation is undertaken with the same care and precision as surgery on the living patient. In the event of multi-organ donation, two or three surgical teams may be called in from transplant hospitals elsewhere in the country. An anaesthetist is present to help support the donor's circulation during the operation. He or she also administers drugs to prevent any sudden movements – caused by lingering spinal reflexes – which could impede the surgery.

The first task, in a complicated procedure which may take anything from four to six hours, is to check the internal organs for any trace of previously undetected damage or disease. The ventilator is then disconnected, the circulating blood is drained off and the organs are flushed through with a cold preservation fluid while still in the donor body. The required organs can then be taken in order: heart, lungs (or occasionally heart and lungs en bloc), liver, kidneys and pancreas. As each organ is removed, it is immersed in a preserving fluid and packed into a container in a cocoon of crushed ice. Time is of the essence with the heart and lungs especially – these must be grafted within four to six hours – and surgical teams are under pressure to return to their various hospitals, where the recipients are waiting, as quickly as possible.

The surgeons ensure that the surgical wound is closed with stitches, just as it would be after any operation. Then the last offices – the cleansing and preparation of the body ready for its removal by the funeral director – are carried out by the theatre staff and one of the SNODs. Afterwards, the body is either returned to the ICU – where some people may care to take leave of a loved one – or to the hospital's chapel of rest. Or, where there has been no request to view, the body is taken straight to the mortuary.

In due course, one of the SNODs writes to the bereaved family with news of the various recipients who have benefited from the donation. Also, they may encourage the recipients to write their own letters of thanks.[1] Their letters are forwarded from the SNODs' office so that the anonymity of donors and recipients is preserved.

---

1. A collection of these letters has recently been published by the Royal College of Physicians under the heading Thankyou for Life.

Chapter 3

Turning Back the Clock

Most people coming into contact with organ donation, whether by signing up as a donor or through bereavement, will be expecting the brainstem death scenario described in the previous chapter. Few people realise that for some while now transplant teams have been turning the clock back more than thirty years. Faced with the fact that the supply of heartbeating donors is a dwindling resource – one which is never going to meet the continually rising demand for organs – they have gone back to the earlier practice of identifying non-ventilated donors. These include patients dying elsewhere in the hospital, not just in intensive care.

Originally, all organs for transplantation were from patients who had been certified dead in the traditional way – that is, after their hearts had stopped. Then came the first formal recognition, by the Harvard Medical Committee in 1968, that death ensues from irreversible damage to the brainstem. This was followed in the UK by the introduction of brainstem death protocols in 1976, yielding a supply of potential donors whose organs could be kept in optimum condition for grafting. The earlier practice of non-heartbeating donation was largely discontinued.

Of course, there never were going to be enough beating-heart donors to keep pace with the spiralling waiting lists and transplanters soon looked for alternatives to make good the organ shortfall. One initiative, pioneered at the Royal Devon and Exeter Hospital in 1988, was elective ventilation: the use of artificial ventilation in comatose patients who were close to death from severe brain damage. This uniquely British practice was designed to ensure that dying patients' organs remained viable for transplantation and, nineteen months after its introduction, the Royal Devon and Exeter reported an increase in kidney donors of more than 80 per cent. Some other hospitals introduced elective ventilation, which at the time had the approval of a number of eminent bodies, including the British Transplantation Society, the British Medical Association and several of the royal colleges.

However, the practice remained highly controversial. For one thing it contravened the common law requirement that medical treatment should be carried out for the benefit of the patient, not that of some third party. Also, there was the perceived risk that gravely ill patients, taken into intensive care, might not die but instead survive with catastrophic deficits, possibly even becoming vegetative (although no such cases were ever reported). At length, having taken legal advice, the Department of Health banned elective ventilation in October 1994.

The following year specialists attending an international meeting in the Dutch city of Maastricht set out to formalise the revival of non-heartbeating donation by agreeing a classification of circumstances in which it could take place. The Maastricht classification (which was later modified) groups potential donors in two broad categories: uncontrolled and controlled. The former includes: those who are dead on arrival at hospital; those seen to undergo cardiac arrest before reaching hospital but who cannot be resuscitated within ten minutes by trained personnel; and brainstem-dead patients whose hearts stop before the relevant tests are carried out. Controlled cases involve patients who are expected to go into cardiac arrest shortly – mainly people whose injuries are not compatible with survival. Non-heartbeating donation is now referred to as donation after cardiac death (DCD).

Almost anyone dying in hospital can be a potential organ or tissue donor, but in practice by far the most common DCD scenario has proved to be where, in the accident and emergency department (A & E) or intensive care unit (ICU), a patient's brain has been irreparably damaged by injury or illness and death is inevitable. So in fact the diagnoses leading to death in the controlled DCD situation are similar to those found in the brainstem-dead population: mainly subarachnoid haemorrhage, head injury or brain damage caused by oxygen starvation. Many of these patients will die in intensive care without fulfilling the criteria for brainstem death.

In the past when a suitable patient went into cardiac arrest, only kidneys were donated. This was because kidneys tolerate a longer period without oxygen than other organs. Now, however, with a number of technical advances helping to keep organs viable for grafting, the liver, lungs and pancreas may also be taken from controlled donors. Lungs are proving most suitable for DCD, since they remain viable so long as they can be kept inflated (even for a while after the circulation has ceased).

The key consideration with DCD is warm ischaemic time: the length of time in which organs remain in the body once the heart has stopped pumping blood and before they have been cooled with preservation fluid. Ischaemic damage to organs means that graft function could be delayed or that the transplanted organ will never work (primary non-function). This is less of a problem with kidneys, where there is the fall-back of dialysis and which in any case remain viable longer, but it is critical with other organs. Clearly, if a transplanted liver or set of lungs fail to work, the recipient dies unless they are given a further transplant.

At present, hearts do not routinely feature in DCD because they can only be reliably restarted if they have been stopped artificially. However, various techniques are being tried to safeguard the viability of donated hearts. For instance, the first ever DCD heart transplant took place in Germany in 2005, where the heartbeat was preserved by circulating blood through an extracorporeal (outside the body) perfusion device. In 2007, the first published account of non-heartbeating donation being used for heart transplants in children involved three infants treated at the Denver Children's Hospital in Colorado. All three babies survived, despite being at high risk of death, and were reported to be alive three and a half years later.

The logistics of DCD vary with the circumstances. In cases where further treatment would be futile, there is a clear separation between the decision to withdraw treatment and the request for donation. Treatment withdrawal is not uncommon in acute hospitals: it occurs in 12 per cent of all ICU admissions and is associated with 50 per cent of deaths in the critical care setting. When DCD is a possibility it is the clinical team caring for the patient who make this decision while transplant personnel 'remain discreet' (to quote one hospital's protocol) until the heart has stopped.

The SNOD meanwhile helps to verify the patient's suitability as a donor and in due course meets the family to discuss donation. If consent is given, he or she talks the family through the various procedures that will be necessary, including blood sampling (for crossmatching) and, once death has been certified, flushing the kidneys through with cold preservative fluid by means of a hollow tube called a cannula, which is inserted into a blood vessel in the groin; a second cannula is inserted to drain fluid away. Occasionally, in a move sanctioned by the Human Tissue Act 2004, steps may be taken to protect the organs before relatives can be contacted, but donation will be subject to consent. Families can withdraw consent at any point and transplant teams will stand down.

The medical staff or SNOD will explain that it sometimes takes quite a while for death to occur following withdrawal of treatment. If there is an appreciable delay, the organs will have deteriorated to the point where they are no longer viable for grafting, although tissues such as corneas, bone or heart valves may still be taken. Donation may also have to be abandoned owing to manpower problems or a shortage of theatre time. The relatives are warned that, once the heart stops, there will be a delay of five minutes before death is certified. If any other organs are to be taken in addition to the kidneys, the donor is taken swiftly to the operating theatre for the retrieval surgery.

The stand-off period is to ensure that the patient does not suddenly show signs of revival, as occasionally happens. Cardiac death is defined as the irreversible loss of heartbeat, breathing and responsiveness. The problem is with 'irreversible' and the lurking fear here is the Lazarus phenomenon. Confusingly, this term has been used in other situations, but in this context it is defined as the unexpected return of spontaneous circulation after resuscitation has been discontinued. In other words, against all odds the heart starts to beat again.

Cardiopulmonary resuscitation (CPR) is continued until the patient recovers or, when there is no response, until it is considered inappropriate to continue – the assumption being that, after a considerable time without oxygen, the brain will have been irreparably damaged. When CPR ceases, death soon intervenes. However, in rare cases – and mostly within ten minutes of stopping CPR – the patient is seen to revive spontaneously.

The Lazarus phenomenon, which has only ever been described after CPR has been abandoned, was first mentioned in the medical literature in 1982, although the actual term was only coined, from the biblical raising of Lazarus (St John's Gospel, Chapter 11), more than a decade later. The Lazarus phenomenon is thought to be very rare, although it is likely that most cases go unreported. By 2002, only twenty-eight cases had been recorded in the medical literature and of these patients, eight returned home without brain damage.

The most memorable of several well-publicised examples is that of a 45-year-old man who collapsed with a heart attack close to the renowned Pitié-Salpêtrière Hospital in Paris in January 2008. Efforts were made to revive him at the scene and resuscitation was continued in the hospital for ninety minutes, apparently to no avail. He was certified dead and, as surgeons were preparing to remove his organs, a pulse returned and he began to breathe unaided. After a long period in intensive care, he recovered and eventually was able to walk and talk. In its special report on the episode, the French hospital's ethics committee confirmed that other clinicians had admitted witnessing similar cases: 'Participants conceded that these were exceptional cases but ones that were nevertheless seen in the course of a career.'

So, whereas brainstem death is unequivocal, cardiac arrest is not necessarily the end of the story. In fact, this issue proved such a vexed one that, in October 2008, the Academy of Medical Royal Colleges published a new code for the diagnosis and confirmation of death. This sets out a standardised protocol, including bedside checks for irreversible cardiorespiratory failure, backed up, in the hospital setting, by evidence from monitoring equipment such as a continuous 'flatline' on the electrocardiogram (ECG, a recording of the heart's electrical activity).

Even so, there remain a number of problems with DCD. For one thing, the business of identifying and maintaining a potential donor in A & E can turn into a logistical nightmare. Until recently it was forbidden even to move a patient who was expected to die imminently. It is often said that, already overstretched, these departments have neither the space nor the experience to handle organ donation. This is likely to prove a singular challenge for the growing number of organ donation champions (formerly known as clinical leads for organ donation, CLODs) appearing in A & E.

There is concern, too, about the potential conflict of interest between the decision to withdraw treatment and the demands of transplantation, particularly with recent moves to 'embed' SNODs within critical care units. Also, many hospital staff are bothered by the fact that, given the time it takes to mobilise an organ retrieval team, withdrawal of treatment will be scheduled to suit the transplanters rather than the potential donor and his or her family. The feeling is that the patient's final hours are being stage-managed according to the needs of organ donation.

There is also an issue of informed consent, because it is true to say that there has been no clear and specific attempt to advise the public of the return to DCD or to explain what it is all about. For instance, the official organ donation website (www.organdonation.nhs.uk) does not go into detail, even in its Q & A section. At best, under 'Donor care' it refers the reader to an outdated publication, the 'UK hospital policy for organ and tissue donation' (2003). This in turn suggests that one should refer to individual hospital policies for further information. Anyone pursuing the subject further will find that not all these policies are available to the public and those which are show considerable variation.

In November 2008, the *British Journal of Anaesthesia* described DCD as the 'most contentious topic' within the UK intensive care community in the previous five years and it is no secret that a number of units have notified NHSBT (formerly UK Transplant) that they do not want to be involved in the practice. Even the massively influential Organ Donation Taskforce report (see Chapter 4), which came out in January 2008, acknowledged that there are outstanding problems and that 'currently the legal position with regard to non-heartbeating donation is unclear, in particular because it differs across the UK'. It concedes that these problems require urgent resolution so as to give hospital staff 'a clear and unambiguous framework of good practice'. One outcome of the report has been the establishment of an independent donation ethics group, which will no doubt ponder the ethical issues raised by cadaver donation.

Meanwhile, the Department of Health has published (November 2009) a Web document entitled 'Legal issues relevant to transplantation', which gives its view of action that can lawfully be taken prior to death to support DCD. 'The intention is that those working in this area will be able to use it to draw up more detailed guidance to support clinical practice.' In other words, clinical staff are left to work out their own salvation.

What is interesting about the DoH report is its insistence that, once it is established that a dying patient would want to donate, all the earlier constraints, to do with such things as taking blood tests, giving drugs to strengthen the heartbeat, increasing oxygen settings, introducing supportive drugs and fluids and even moving the patient to a more convenient area, are all now permissible in the person's 'best interests'; so long as they do not cause harm or distress. It remains to be seen how families will react to having their loved ones shunted between departments and to the inevitable delays in withdrawing treatment.

At present, time is the limiting factor. Initiatives being developed following acceptance of the Taskforce recommendations will only reach their full potential when there are fail-safe methods for limiting ischaemic damage. A number of centres are working to maximise the yield of organs from DCD, with strategies ranging from adding oxygen to preservative fluid, to connecting the donor to an external apparatus which circulates oxygenated blood (extracorporeal membrane oxygenation, ECMO, as in the German heart transplant mentioned earlier), to keep the organs viable. Especially promising is an experimental device, developed by scientists at Oxford University, which has been used to keep livers viable outside the body for more than seventy-two hours. Clinical trials are under way and the hope is that the technique can be extended to other organs.

So far as hearts are concerned, two British hospitals, Papworth near Cambridge and Harefield in Middlesex, have been involved in the European trial of a portable warm blood perfusion system which provides the donor heart with a continuous blood flow. The Organ Care System consists of a sterile chamber in which the beating heart is kept at a constant temperature while oxygenated blood withdrawn from the donor is pumped into it, mimicking natural circulation. In this way, the heart can be maintained in good condition for up to twelve hours. According to the US manufacturer, it contains 'novel technologies that simulate the conditions of the human body'.

The system, first used in the UK in the summer of 2006, could boost the number of transplants by cutting down wastage of donated hearts. Meanwhile, the manufacturer is hoping to apply the same technology to other organs intended for grafting. It could also, they say, enhance the use of 'marginal' organs – that is, ones which are less than ideal – by allowing a surgeon time 'to potentially resuscitate the organ *ex vivo* to build up its energy stores'.

Certainly DCD is here to stay. Research has shown that, while kidneys taken in this situation may be slow to function, the results after five years are as good as transplants from beating-heart donors. This was confirmed in August 2010 by research carried out jointly by specialists from NHS Blood and Transplant and Addenbrooke's Hospital in 2010. They predicted that DCD will have become the predominant source of kidneys for grafting by the year 2015. There is less experience with other organs, but early signs are that liver, pancreas and lung transplants using DCD compare well with those from ventilated donors.

In 2001 only 42 DCD kidney transplants were carried out in the UK. By the year 2009–10, the figure had risen to 329. During this same year – the latest for which figures are available – DCD was yielding almost one in six of all solid organs for transplantation.

Chapter 4

A Terrible Dichotomy

Everyone knows about organ transplants and most people seem to think they are a good thing. But still, after more than half a century of increasing transplant activity, there remains this terrible dichotomy: the fact that, while more than 90 per cent of the population supports organ donation, when permission to donate is sought from people facing bereavement, almost half refuse. There is considerable regional variation in the refusal rate, ranging from a low of 30 per cent in the south-east generally to 49 per cent in London, but overall our refusal rate is one of the worst in Europe.

This means that, with more than 8,000 very sick patients on the active waiting list for transplantation, there are never enough organs to meet their needs. This figure understates the position since access to waiting lists for livers, hearts and lungs are restricted to some extent because of the chronic shortage of donor organs. The true need is likely to be for at least 50 per cent more transplants than are currently available and figures will continue to spiral out of sight because of Britain's changing demographics. The population is continuing to increase and so, too, are the proportion of elderly people and the percentage of ethnic minorities, some of whom are particularly vulnerable to health problems leading to organ failure.

Almost all the principal conditions requiring solid organ transplants are increasing, including cardiomyopathy (heart), cystic fibrosis (lungs) and a number of liver conditions, especially alcoholic cirrhosis.

End-stage kidney failure is rising at a rate of 2 per cent each year and a particular concern is the continuing increase in Types 1 and 2 diabetes which, of course, can lead to kidney failure. Meanwhile, each year more than 1,000 waiting recipients – an average of 3 a day – die before they can be transplanted. Currently, some 10–15 per cent of people on the waiting list for a liver – the second most frequently transplanted organ after the kidney – are dying before an organ becomes available.

Most organs for grafting come from a relatively small population of ventilated patients who have been confirmed brainstem-dead (see Chapter 2), many of whom have the potential to become multi-organ donors. However, for some years the number of brainstem deaths – which represent less than 1 per cent of all deaths in the UK – has been falling. This decline is mainly owing to improvements in road safety – especially the introduction of seat belts – and advances in neurosurgical care. There was some consternation in transplant circles when it was found that the annual rate of donation had fallen by 14 per cent (from 739 to 633) between the years 2000 and 2006. So, the size of the donor pool has dwindled. Currently, little more than 600 heartbeating donors are becoming available each year.

Another issue has been the failure of staff to identify potential donors. Part of the problem here is unfamiliarity since, for many of the UK's 250–300 acute hospitals, brainstem death is an infrequent event. The Intensive Care Society's estimate is that an ICU in an average-sized general hospital may have only 5 to 10 potential heartbeating donors in a year. The largest units with neurosurgical facilities will have a maximum of 25–30 a year. The potential donor audit pioneered by UK Transplant has revealed that a significant number of patients for whom brainstem death is a possible diagnosis do not undergo tests for this condition. Also, in 15 per cent of cases where brainstem death is confirmed there is no record of the families being approached for organ donation.

A number of initiatives have been developed to increase the number of referrals, including training days and workshops for medical and nursing staff. An early innovator here was the Royal Bolton Hospital, which as far back as 2002 brought in a raft of measures in order to increase donation. These included scheduling staff study days, the introduction of 'required referral' of potential donors in the ICU and the amalgamation of donor and bereavement services.

All this brought about a sea change in beliefs and attitudes. Over time, Bolton achieved a 100 per cent referral rate for both non-heartbeating and heartbeating donation. The consent rate for solid organ donation shot up to 90 per cent and the number of relatives giving permission for tissue retrieval went from 6 in 2002 to 246 in 2008. This remarkable effort pre-empted the recommendations that would be reached by the government-appointed Organ Donation Taskforce (see below) and in fact it has been said that if all hospitals were achieving organ donation at the rate of the 20 per cent of top-performing centres there would be 40 per cent more organs available for transplants.

There is some evidence that the consent rate for organ donation is higher when a collaborative approach is taken to requesting. Researchers at the John Radcliffe Hospital in Oxford combed various literature to find out what influenced people's decisions. One of these (mostly American) studies recorded: 53 per cent of relatives giving consent when a doctor or nurse alone made the request; 62 per cent agreeing when a transplant co-ordinator asked; and 72 per cent allowed organs to be used when a doctor and a transplant co-ordinator made a joint approach. The John Radcliffe team found: 'The two factors that had the largest effect on consent rates were the person making the request and the timing of this conversation.' Perhaps not surprisingly, family members are much more likely to refuse if they are asked for organs at the same time as being told that their relative is brainstem-dead.

With waiting lists for transplant at an all-time high, the transplant community has responded to the chronic shortfall in two ways: by eking out the available organs, such as using split livers, or by casting around for new sources. For example, there have been suggestions across the developed world that organs should be taken from patients in a permanent vegetative state (PVS), a condition in which the patient never regains consciousness. A survey of physicians in the US, where there are thought to be up to 25,000 such cases, revealed that almost two thirds believed that it would be ethical to use the organs of patients in PVS for transplantation.

In the UK a short-lived innovation was 'elective ventilation': targeting certain patients – mostly stroke victims – who had been admitted to hospital with no chance of survival and, with relatives' consent, transferring them to intensive care to be ventilated so that they could become donors. This scheme, pioneered at the Royal Devon and Exeter Hospital in 1988, was taken up by a number of hospitals, enabling the identification of some patients who would not otherwise have become donors. However, in the light of legal opinion that elective ventilation contravenes the law, the practice was discontinued in 1994.

Less controversial has been the growing use of non-ventilated donors, who were identified for what is known as donation after cardiac death (DCD). These may be patients anywhere in the hospital who are on the brink of death but who cannot be resuscitated successfully. An increasing number of A & E departments in particular are co-operating in this mode of donation, pinpointing patients who can contribute not only solid organs but also other tissues.

Another tactic is the use of expanded criteria donation (ECD) or even extreme expanded criteria donation (X-ECD), yielding what are known as 'marginal' organs – those which are elderly, diseased or damaged in some way. The use of deceased donors more than fifty years old has increased by 135 per cent in the past decade or so and it is well known that kidneys and livers are sometimes taken from people in their seventies and eighties. The only absolute contra-indications to organ donation are: known infection with HIV, the AIDS virus; known or suspected Creutzfeldt-Jakob disease (CJD), the human form of BSE; and the presence of some cancers.

From time to time organs from cancer victims, suicides, drinkers, drug users and smokers have been used for transplants. A number of notorious cases have come to light in the UK, including that of the 31-year-old soldier who, in February 2008, died from lung cancer after receiving the lungs of a fifty-a-day smoker. A 37-year-old man who had suffered heart problems since childhood underwent a heart transplant at the same hospital five months later, but he never regained consciousness. The grafted heart, which had failed to restart, had a hole in it which had been repaired beforehand. It had come from a donor who had hanged himself; he had been a smoker, had used drugs from time to time and had been tested for HIV.

The full details of this case only came to light at the inquest and there have been other instances where substandard organs have been transplanted without the knowledge of the recipients or their relatives. On the other hand, many surgeons go to great lengths to explain the situation, pointing out the risk/benefit trade-off between accepting a marginal organ or turning it down and having to face continued deterioration and, in some cases, certain death. In 2007, a surgeon in the US notched up a dubious first by removing the heart of a deceased heart recipient and re-transplanting it into another patient.

Also battling hopelessly long waiting lists, surgeons at a hospital in Ehime, Japan, nearly twenty years ago began taking diseased kidneys from living patients, 'repairing' them on the workbench and grafting them into waiting recipients. In Brisbane, a team at the Princess Alexandra Hospital reported on a series of forty-three patients, all of whom were more than 60 years of age, who had received 'repaired' kidneys. After three and a half years four of them had died, all from conditions unrelated to the grafts. According to the Australian team, ten would have been expected to die each year if they had remained on dialysis.

Lungs are most susceptible to damage around the time of brainstem death and only about 15–20 per cent of those offered for transplantation are viable. For this reason researchers are working on ways and means to salvage more of them for use. Particularly promising is a new technique, developed in Canada and Sweden, for 'reconditioning' donated lungs by means of something called an *ex vivo* lung perfusion (EVLP) system. This involves placing the donated lungs into a chamber and then infusing them with a restorative solution of nutrients, steroids and antibiotics. The hope is that the EVLP system could increase the use of donor lungs by 30–40 per cent.

Canadian researchers are also experimenting with the addition of gene therapy to the use of EVLP to reclaim damaged lungs. The gene in question, known as IL-10, is present in both human and animal cells and plays a part in inhibiting the immune response. The IL-10 gene is injected into the donor lungs contained in a viral vector. After about six hours it is seen to begin producing the anti-inflammatory proteins that will counter the earlier damage. Donor lungs undergoing both EVLP and gene therapy showed significantly improved function, with the boosted IL-10 effect found to last for up to thirty days. The Toronto team believe that ultimately the same principle could be applied to other donor organs.

While the use of marginal donors is controversial, the ideal donor is becoming increasingly rare. For one thing, whereas traumatic brain injury used to be the commonest cause of brainstem death, today the main cause of this condition is brain haemorrhage. Now, instead of organs coming from young, fit individuals, they are more likely to come from older, sicker stroke victims. In this country the average age of cadaver donors has risen to forty-six. So, the argument goes, if transplant surgeons were to wait for perfect organs, waiting lists would be even longer.

There is evidence that transplants using old kidneys are associated with a higher rate of graft loss and even death of the patient. Nephrologists at Stanford University in California devised a way of comparing the performance of the older transplanted kidney by testing the function of the glomerulus, the network of capillaries which is the site of primary filtration of waste products. They found that, at three months post-transplant, kidneys which had come from donors over the age of 55 performed only 70 per cent as well as those from donors less than 40 years of age. Older kidneys contained less than half the normal quantity of functioning glomeruli and these were seen to be swollen – an indication of overwork.

UK centres could be among the first to use a new test, developed at Glasgow University, to ascertain the biological rather than chronological age of a kidney. The researchers isolated a genetic factor which showed a strong link with declining kidney function, demonstrating that biological age is a more reliable indicator of the organ's viability than is the chronological age of the donor.

The most reliable source of healthy organs are live donors (see Chapter 5), an increasing number of whom are coming forward to offer organs for transplantation. The number of living donor kidney transplants has soared over the last decade or so – to a total of 1,037 for the year 2009–10 – and now accounts for more than a third of all kidney transplants. Living donors can also contribute parts of other organs.

For years, the main hope for whittling away at the refusal rate has been to persuade more people to sign up to the NHS Organ Donor Register (ODR), the computerised service set up in October 1994 to enable people to record their willingness to donate their organs in the event of their death. By the end of June 2011, upwards of 18 million people – some 29 per cent of the UK population – had signed the register.

A particular concern is to secure increased commitment from various ethnic groups, in particular South Asians and Afro-Caribbeans, who make up 8 per cent of the UK population and who are three to four times more likely than Caucasians to develop kidney failure. Already, 13 per cent of patients needing new kidneys are Asian and 7 per cent are black. Together, they make up 23 per cent of the waiting list for kidney transplant and the estimate is that, within a few years, black and Asian groups may account for half the patients on dialysis in parts of the UK with large ethnic communities. As it is, the refusal rate for organ donation soars to 75 per cent among non-whites and only about 3 per cent of cadaver donors come from these ethnic groups.

In 2004, UK Transplant (since subsumed into NHS Blood and Transplant, NHSBT) commissioned a twelve-month study of families who had refused consent for donation. Researchers from Southampton University were able to pinpoint a number of the factors involved in families' decision-making, including: the timing, manner and content of the donation discussion; people's views about keeping the body intact; and their need to be with the dying person and witness the end of life 'represented by cessation of the heartbeat'.

According to UKT: 'Protecting the body, which related to keeping the body whole and intact, was the most frequently recurring theme underpinning a decision not to donate. Fifteen participants said that they could not bear the thought of their deceased relative being "cut up" ...'

A year earlier the British Organ Donor Society (BODY) had commissioned the same team to investigate the experiences of bereaved adults with whom donation had been discussed. This highlighted the difficulty which shocked and grieving people have in getting to grips with the notion of brainstem death. The authors felt that understanding death as certified by brainstem testing is a key factor in deciding whether or not to allow donation to go ahead and has been shown to 'have an impact on subsequent grief'. Whether in the DCD setting relatives will be any more willing to consent to donation remains to be seen.

More recently the NHSBT carried out an online survey to try to establish why people fail to sign up to the ODR and two main reasons emerged: concern about the level of respect shown to the dead person's body and uncertainty as to whether doctors would make every possible effort to save someone who had been identified as a potential donor. Many respondents wanted more information about what happens to the body after death. The NHSBT found that the most common reason for not wanting to register is to avoid having to think about dying.

Those who do get as far as ringing the ODR line mention a number of concerns, including how donation might affect funeral arrangements and whether the body will be disfigured after the organs are retrieved. Staff manning the ODR line say many callers don't want to give permission for corneas to be taken 'because they say they want to be able to see where they're going when they die'. In contrast, a lady whose daughter had died in circumstances which precluded solid organ transplantation drew comfort from donating the corneas. She hoped that 'whoever received them would see the world through the same rosy glow' that her daughter had. This concern about the eyes is widespread. Many bereaved relatives and more than a million people who have put themselves on the ODR have held back on donating eyes. Many people fear disfigurement, although the cosmetic effect, with a prosthesis inserted following enucleation, is probably better than the sunken appearance of the closed eyes which develops some time after death.

It is because of the deepening crisis in organ supply that a system which has developed piecemeal over the years is now being forced to undergo seismic change. This was set in train in January 2008 with publication of a report, 'Organs for Transplants', by the Organ Donation Taskforce, which had been set up by the government to look into the obstacles to donation. Unequivocal in its findings, the Taskforce pointed to 'systems failure' as being responsible for the current situation.

This report highlighted a number of key issues needing attention, including the frenetic multitasking required of donor transplant co-ordinators (since renamed specialist nurses in organ donation, SNODs), who are the people responsible for making transplants happen and also for the care of the bereaved families. Until very recently, each cadaver donation would involve a single donor co-ordinator attending the donor hospital from the time of referral to the last offices – often a continuous stretch of more than twenty-four hours. Organ retrieval surgery and last offices alone can take up to six hours. The working practices of these nurses – most of them highly specialised – were 'considered unsustainable'.

By way of rationalisation, the Taskforce recommended a significant increase in the number of SNODs – from the 120 or so then in post – and for this enhanced workforce to be brought under the wing of the Organ Donation and Transplantation Directorate (a division of

NHSBT), which would become responsible for recruitment, training and management. The idea was for three SNODs to be available to attend each organ donation: one to work with the family and the other two to manage the awesome logistics. The Taskforce reckoned that a vastly improved donor co-ordination service could boost the consent rate to at least 70 per cent over five years.

Organ retrieval arrangements were also found to be overstretched. Most retrieval surgery takes place at night in unfamiliar hospitals and often involves specialist teams from several centres. Delays are commonplace and these cause distress to families and disruption to host hospitals, as well as putting the stability of donors at risk, which threatens the viability of the organs. The Taskforce recommended establishment of a countrywide network of dedicated retrieval teams which would provide round-the-clock availability.

Altogether, the Taskforce made fourteen recommendations in the belief that implementation of these – to a great extent already going ahead – would create a 'structured and systematic approach' to organ donation in the UK. The estimate was that these measures would result in a 50 per cent increase in organ donation rates within five years, resulting in an additional 1,200 transplants per annum with at least 1,000 lives a year saved and greatly improved quality of life for many people. Above all, the report urged, all parts of the NHS should 'embrace' organ donation as a usual event and part of end-of-life care.

In a subsequent report, 'The potential impact of an opt-out system for organ donation in the UK', published in November 2008, the Taskforce managed to resist pressure to come down in favour of what is known as 'presumed consent'. This is in effect a reversal of the present system, in that it would mean that organs could be taken from potential donors if they had not opted out; that is, registered an objection to donation. The transplant community, patient groups and successive governments have resisted this over the years but recently there has been growing pressure for an opt-out system.

Advocates point to a recent analysis of twenty-eight countries showing that those with presumed consent have higher donation rates than those without it. Spain, for instance, has the highest recorded rate in the world at 31.5 per million of the population (compared to the UK's 12.8 per million). However, the introduction of presumed consent in Spain in 1979 did little for the first decade and real gains only came with the rationalisation of the donor co-ordination system. In the UK many people feel, as the Taskforce members did, that the introduction of presumed consent could be counterproductive, causing a drop in donations.

A disturbing aspect of the organ shortage has been the runaway growth of a global market in human organs and tissues. A flagrant example came to light when racketeers took bones from the body of the British broadcaster Alistair Cooke, which had been lying in a funeral parlour in New York City. Cooke was 95 years old when he died of cancer in 2004. The racketeer in chief, a former dentist who ran a New Jersey biotech company, admitted plundering some 1,800 cadavers (supplied by funeral directors) for body parts which were then sold on.

A medical anthropologist at the University of Berkeley, California, Nancy Scheper-Hughes, had set up an organisation five years earlier known as Organs Watch to investigate allegations of medical abuse in the harvesting, distribution and transplantation of organs. She and her team chronicled evidence from four continents of what she called 'human strip mining of the dead for usable body parts'. They also documented cases where organs had been taken from the living, often without their knowledge, and of the abduction of children for their organs. Typically the Berkeley team found exploitation of the poor, mostly in Eastern Europe and the Third World, for the benefit of affluent recipients in the West.

In Britain it is well known that many transplant tourism recipients suffer a higher rate of ill effects and even fatalities than patients treated here. In mid-2006, a Birmingham kidney specialist carried out a survey of local patients who, tired of lingering indefinitely on dialysis, had acquired kidneys in India the previous year. One in eight had died within weeks of surgery and two thirds had suffered post-operative complications.

By 2008, the World Health Organisation (WHO) estimate was that some 10 per cent of all transplants worldwide involve unacceptable or illegal activities. In the spring of that year delegates from seventy-eight countries met in Istanbul to agree a ban on transplant tourism. The 'Declaration of Istanbul on Organ Trafficking and Transplant Tourism', issued in July 2008, urged the disqualification of transplant surgeons involved in illegal transactions. In Britain, North America and all member countries of the EU it has for some years been illegal to trade in human organs for transplantation.

It is hard to see how there will ever be sufficient organs to meet the rising demand. There may be more than 18 million people on the ODR, but the fact remains that only a tiny percentage of them will ever donate. To do so, one has to be in hospital, preferably in an ICU or A & E, be free of cancer and infection and have relatives readily available to give permission. No less a figure than the National Clinical Director for Transplantation, Chris Rudge – the transplant 'tsar' – has confirmed that only about 1,500 to 2,000 people a year in this country die in circumstances conducive to organ donation. It is for this reason that researchers are busy pursuing a number of alternatives to transplantation (see Chapter 8).

Chapter 5

The Living Donor

Live donation is not exactly new. Living donors were surrendering one of their kidneys for grafting long before cadaver organs were made available. Now, however, with the queues for organ transplants stretching into infinity, a whole new generation of relatives, friends and sometimes even strangers are coming forward to offer not only kidneys but also lobes or segments of lung, liver, small bowel or pancreas to make good the organ shortfall. Perhaps not surprisingly, more women are volunteering as live donors than men.

The first ever successful kidney transplant took place in Boston, Massachusetts, in 1954, when Ronald Herrick donated a kidney to his very sick identical twin, Richard, who lived for a further eight years. In Britain, the first successful living donor transplant – also a kidney, also between twins – was carried out in Edinburgh in 1961. But it is only in the last decade or so that live donation has become commonplace. The transaction is, of course, most feasible with kidneys and today more than a third of all renal transplants in the UK are performed using kidneys donated by the living.

Given the severe shortage of cadaver organs, there is a strong case to be made for live donation of kidneys. Already, the waiting time for a new kidney is some two and a half to three years; and as much as five years or more for some minority ethnic groups. Moreover, since the incidence of chronic kidney failure will continue to increase, owing to an ageing population and rising lifestyle-associated factors such as hypertension, obesity and, most especially, diabetes, these intervals are likely to become even longer.

There are clear advantages to live donation. For a start, kidneys transplanted from live donation last twice as long as cadaver organs and recipients also live longer. The one-year success rate for a kidney grafted from a living donor is 96 per cent, compared with 93 per cent for one from a deceased donor. Moreover, the average 'lifespan' of a living kidney transplant from a relative is around twelve years, compared with only ten years for a cadaver kidney. A further consideration is that live donation enables patients in chronic renal failure to be transplanted earlier in the course of their disease – possibly before they reach the stage of needing dialysis – and this pre-emptive transplantation has been shown to give significantly better long-term survival.

Naturally, most live donors are relatives or friends of the recipients, although the Human Tissue Act 2004, which came into effect in September 2006, permits so-called 'altruistic' donation from strangers (known as 'good Samaritan' donors in the US). The first of these to be reported, in 2007, was the case of a retired carpenter in Bedfordshire who received a kidney from a nurse in Plymouth. Human Tissue Authority figures show that twenty-two kidney transplants using altruistic donations had been performed by April 2011. Live, unrelated donors are particularly welcome for people whose renal failure is the result of some inherited condition, where other blood relatives either already have or will have the same problem.

People contemplating donation, who must be over 18 years of age, will undergo searching psychological and physical assessments, including laboratory tests and various scans, to ensure both that they are compatible with the intended recipient and that they are completely fit. They are warned beforehand that this rigorous work-up – it may take three months or more – may show up previously undetected conditions. Hospitals stress that the donor is free to change their mind at any point. All parties to live donation – both donor and recipient – are seen by a local assessor who is independent of the health teams involved and who recommends to the Human Tissue Authority that the planned transplant should go ahead.

Tissue type is indicated by 'marker' proteins on the surface of the body's cells. The higher percentage of donor proteins that match those of the intended recipient, the less likelihood there is of rejection. This tissue compatibility is mostly seen in close relatives and, of course, is total in identical twins. Transplants are performed where the tissue match is less than ideal, but a good match is essential for recipients with an unusually large number of circulating antibodies. These highly sensitised patients have usually had previous exposure to 'foreign' tissue, such as an earlier transplant, blood transfusion or pregnancy.

Sometimes, where there is a compatibility problem, a few centres will offer a desensitising programme enabling donors to give a non-matching kidney. This involves treating the recipient with a drug to suppress antibody production and also cleansing his or her blood of potentially destructive antibodies using the techniques known as plasma exchange or antigen-specific immunoadsorption (see following chapter). This ensures that the transplant can go ahead without the risk of instant rejection. Clearly, the risk of rejection is higher in incompatible transplants, but the estimate is that at least 70 per cent would be working a year after surgery (compared with up to 95 per cent after well-matched donation).

The 2004 Act also sanctioned what is known as paired/pooled donation, where a would-be donor and recipient whose tissues are not compatible are matched (anonymously) with another pair in the same situation. Originally it was reckoned that there would need to be a pool of at least 20 or 30, and ideally 50, entries to ensure the identification of some matching pairs. By January 2009 there were 126 pairs registered. The first paired transplant took place in July 2007, with one pair hospitalised in Edinburgh and the other in Cambridge. The two donors were provided with a continuous phone link right up to the point where anaesthesia was induced – simultaneously – in case either of them felt they couldn't go through with it. The donated kidneys were flown between the two centres.

Normally the donor and recipient operations take place simultaneously in adjoining theatres, so as to keep to a minimum what is known as the ischaemic time, that is the time that the kidney is deprived of its blood supply. The operation to remove the kidney (donor nephrectomy) is done either by the traditional open surgery or, increasingly, by the newer technique of laparoscopic ('keyhole') surgery. For technical reasons in each case the left kidney is usually the one to be taken.

The open procedure, which involves a long incision running from the upper abdomen and around the ribs on one side – although some surgeons prefer an abdominal incision – takes about two hours. The kidney is lifted out and flushed through with cold solution to wash out blood and slow metabolism before being taken to the recipient in an adjoining theatre. The donor normally stays in hospital from seven to ten days and full recuperation takes anything from two to three months. There is a newer technique of open mini-incision nephrectomy, developed at the Hammersmith Hospital in west London, which involves only a single 3–5 cm incision (1.25–2 in). The pioneers claim that it is safer and enables faster recovery.

The keyhole procedure (laparoscopic nephrectomy) was pioneered in the US in the early 1990s and brought to the UK more than a decade ago. It involves making three small incisions in the abdomen, two of which are for the instruments; the kidney is withdrawn through the largest, which is usually just below the bikini line. The donor is out of hospital within two to four days and back to full activity after about four to six weeks.

As part of the drive to increase live donation, the transplant community is making laparoscopic donor nephrectomy more widely available. While it often takes longer than the open procedure, it has been shown to have significant advantages, including far less requirement for painkillers, a shorter hospital stay, faster recovery and a much more acceptable cosmetic appearance – with a few inconspicuous marks as opposed to an 18 cm (7 in) scar.

Transplant teams have had sufficient experience of live donation of kidneys to be able to reassure both parties that the risks to the donor are minimal. If one kidney is removed, the other increases slightly in size and capacity. Apart from the usual risks of surgery, such as infection, the most that tends to happen is that, after the operation, some donors have a slight rise in blood pressure and a slight excess of protein in the urine, neither of which is said to be clinically important.

The risk of death for the donor has been estimated at 1 in 3,300 – comparable to the risk of dying in a road accident. In the US, a review of more than 80,000 adult donors undergoing nephrectomy between 1994 and 2009 showed that just 25 had died within ninety days of surgery. Research has shown that in practice people donating kidneys live longer than the general population. This is no doubt owing to the fact that they were found to be fit to start with and, once they have donated, their health is monitored on a yearly basis.

The position is somewhat different for the other (partial) organs recovered from live donors. Live donation of a lobe of the liver is possible because of this organ's amazing powers of regeneration: remove part of the liver and it regrows, virtually to its original size, within weeks. Surgeons in Brisbane were the first to take part of a liver from a live donor, operating on a 28-year-old mother to save her 1-year-old son, in August 1989. Elsewhere, living donor liver transplants were pioneered in the late 1980s, mainly in response to the high death rate among children waiting for new livers. The procedure, which involves grafting the (smaller) left lobe from an adult into a child, is now well established in paediatric centres.

The adult-to-adult procedure was developed in the early 1990s and is now widely practised in the US, Continental Europe and the Far East. In the UK, where just under 700 liver transplants are carried out each year – but one in five patients dies on the waiting list – living donor liver transplantation (LDLT) on the NHS was only sanctioned a few years ago (although one centre had been transplanting private patients). The first NHS adult-to-adult LDLT was carried out at St James's University Hospital in Leeds in June 2007, when a young man of 20 years donated a lobe of his liver to his 57-year-old father. By January 2009, three centres had between them performed ten adult-to-adult live donor transplants.

In general, the donor operation (hepatic lobectomy) takes three to four hours and the length of hospital stay is about two weeks. The National Institute for Health and Clinical Excellence (NICE), in its review of the literature, found that nearly all donors were back to a full range of normal activities within six months of surgery and by this time their livers had regenerated to an average 89 per cent of their original size.

In fact, there are important differences in the risk-benefit ratios in making live donation for adults or children. For children it is the smaller left lobe of the liver which is used. But since the left lobe does not have sufficient liver mass for adults, the right lobe is used in their case. The donor's risk of death when the right lobe is taken is greater than with the left lobe and the problems are more common. All told, the donor's risk of death is between half and one per cent and the rate of complications is upwards of 20 per cent. Various complications have been documented, including bleeding, infection and intestinal problems. There have even been a couple of cases where the donors developed liver failure themselves and had to undergo 'salvage transplants'. In the face of these risks, some transplant surgeons are reluctant to involve live donors.

NICE gave the survival rate of children whose livers were grafted from live donors as 92 per cent, compared to 81 per cent for those receiving cadaver livers. With adult recipients there is no difference in survival between live or cadaver donation.

Interestingly, in Scotland, which had been the first UK region to get the go-ahead for adult LDLT, a programme was set up at the Edinburgh Royal Infirmary in the spring of 2006. However, by September 2007 it was reported that there had been no takers because would-be recipients saw it as being too risky for their loved ones to undergo. It was not until February 2008 that the hospital reported its first live liver transplant but, as the director of the transplant unit said, 'We are delighted that the operation has gone so well ... However, in many ways we would like not to have to perform live donor liver transplantation. The risks are high for both the recipient and the donor and operating on a donor feels different to anything else that we do because the benefit is not to that patient alone.'

There is a rare situation where a living donor can donate their whole liver in what is known as a domino procedure. The donor here would be someone suffering from one of several metabolic disorders which are treated by liver transplantation. Most common of these is familial amyloid neuropathy (FAP), in which an abnormal protein produced by the liver is deposited throughout the body causing severe effects, including paralysis. Removal of the liver, the source of the abnormal protein, stops the disease progressing. However, the function of the liver is in all other respects normal and, since it would be unlikely to cause FAP symptoms in a recipient for thirty years or more, it can be used to save the life of an older person with severe liver disease. Domino liver transplantation was first introduced in Portugal in 1995.

The only centre with any real experience of live pancreas donation is that at the University of Minnesota, where pancreas grafting was pioneered. This operation was developed for patients with Type 1 diabetes and Minnesota claims a number of world firsts in this area, including the first unrelated live donor partial pancreas transplant.

About half the pancreas is removed – the tail end, sometimes along with a kidney – either by open or keyhole surgery. This centre has in the past retrieved insulin-producing islet cells from live donors, to be injected into a recipient's portal vein. However, they claim that islet infusion is not as effective as pancreas transplant in freeing the recipient from insulin dependence.

There are considerable risks to donors providing pancreatic tissue, not least the possibility that they could themselves develop diabetes. Regarded still as being experimental, partial pancreas donation is not thought to be necessary or justified in the UK. The view is that, for the vast majority of people with diabetes, insulin treatment is safer than pancreas transplantation.

Live donation of the small bowel is rare. Small bowel transplantation is performed for patients with irreversible intestinal failure who are kept alive on a mode of artificial feeding called total parenteral nutrition (TPN) and this can give rise to serious, sometimes life-threatening complications. The first successful living related small bowel transplant took place in Germany in 1988. The first attempt in Britain, in Leeds in 1995, featured a mother donating to her 28-year-old daughter but, having suffered several bouts of rejection, the younger woman died from pneumonia eighteen months later.

One of the advantages of live donation is that there is less risk to the recipient of early infection since the donor's bowel can be 'decontaminated' before surgery goes ahead. The segment of small bowel removed for grafting may be up to about 2 m (6.5 ft) in length, but experience has shown that the risks to the donor are relatively low. The ideal donor, of course, is one who is genetically identical to the recipient, an identical twin (or, as in the first such case carried out in Cambridge in 1997, a triplet). This is because there is no need for the immunosuppressive regimen – especially powerful in small bowel transplantation – which leaves the recipient exposed to a high risk of infection and of certain cancers.

Live lung donation is arguably even more controversial because here the recipient – whose diseased lungs are removed – receives the right lower lobe from one donor and the left lower lobe from another. One study of 123 recipients grafted from live donors showed 70 per cent survival after one year, 54 per cent after three years and 45 per cent after five years; infection was the main cause of death. There is little information on the fate of people sacrificing part of a lung, although about 20 per cent are found to have at least one problem post-operatively. One study showed that donors' lungs 'did not work as well as they did before the operation', but there have been no reports of deaths.

The only situation in which a living person can donate a heart for transplantation is when surgeons decide it is more effective to perform a combined heart-lung transplant for a patient with lung disease. This person's healthy heart is then grafted into a cardiac patient in a domino procedure. In practice, only a few heart-lung transplants are performed each year and so the domino potential is severely limited.

Live donation has been attacked by some as contravening the Hippocratic oath – 'First, do no harm' – and in fact in 1987 no less a body than the British Transplantation Society approved a Council of Europe ruling which urged that removal of organs from living donors should, where possible, be 'gradually eliminated'. The measures being implemented following the recommendations of the Organ Donation Taskforce (see previous chapter) may ease the pressure, but the end of live donation is nowhere in sight.

Chapter 6

The Treatment of Choice

The experience of patients listed for transplant varies with the circumstances. One thing the majority will all have in common is a nail-bitingly long wait. At present, average waiting times for cadaver organs for adults are: about five months for livers; six months for hearts; almost eighteen months for lungs; and, with queues vastly longer than for the other organs, more than three and a half years for kidneys (which is why live donation is becoming increasingly common). Urgent cases take priority and some of these – for instance, patients in acute liver failure – may be comatose in hospital before their surgery.

Another common experience is what is known as a 'bad call' – being called into hospital for a transplant which then for some reason or other does not materialise. One youngster from Lanarkshire, suffering a hereditary heart condition, had to endure five bad calls before finally being transplanted. This kind of experience can be so nerve-wracking that patients who have had a run of bad calls have been known to take themselves off the list. Many would-be recipients – an estimated three a day in the UK – die waiting for a transplant; many more are taken off the active waiting list when they pass the point of no return, becoming too ill to withstand major surgery.

For a glimpse into the recipient experience, this chapter details the events surrounding transplantation of the kidney, the most sought after of the solid organs. By 2009, there were some 45,000 people in the UK with established kidney failure who were being maintained on some form of renal replacement therapy (RRT). Roughly half of these had kidney grafts. The rest, many of them awaiting transplantation, were kept going on some form of dialysis. In addition, there were thousands more patients with deteriorating renal function who would become candidates for RRT at some time in the future.

In fact, nature has endowed human beings with a generous overcapacity of kidney function, which is why many people with only one kidney remain healthy. So generous is the margin that, with skilled care, it is possible for the patient in chronic renal failure to survive without RRT almost to the final stages of their disease. Dialysis or transplantation only become imperative when kidney function has fallen to less than 10 per cent of normal. However, with the increasing use of live donors, some patients whose renal decline is inexorable are opting for pre-emptive transplantation so as to avoid having to undergo dialysis. Patients on waiting lists are two to three times more likely to die than those who receive new kidneys.

Transplantation is widely acknowledged as the treatment of choice for end-stage renal failure, with one-year graft survival rates of up to 96 per cent for living donor cases and 93 per cent for cadaveric grafts. It is also cost-effective according to the government-appointed Organ Donation Taskforce report ,'Organs for transplant' (January 2008), which gave the average annual cost of dialysis as £23,177 per person, compared with an initial £42,025 for a kidney transplant plus £6,500 a year in maintenance costs.

There is a small minority of renal patients who are unsuitable for transplantation. It is not appropriate, for instance, for those with: chronic infection; recent cancer; other life-threatening disease elsewhere than in the kidneys; or some renal disease with a high incidence of recurrence. Active peptic ulcer disease has to be treated successfully before the patient can be considered for a transplant. Rarely, a combined liver-kidney graft may be proposed for someone who also has liver disease.

In many ways the kidney is ideal for grafting. For a start it is a paired organ, which means it can be acquired from either a living or a cadaver donor. Conveniently for surgeons its blood supply is usually simple, making it relatively easy to 'plumb in'. Also, once the blood supply is established, more often than not a grafted kidney begins producing urine on the operating table – gratifying evidence that it is still in good condition.

The allocation of organs is based on what is known as donor compatibility: the establishment of points of agreement between the tissues of the person donating the kidney (whether living or dead) and the would-be recipient. This is done so as to minimise the chances of rejection. Compatibility is determined in three stages: blood grouping, tissue typing and crossmatching.

Blood grouping is as necessary for transplantation as it is for blood transfusions, since the use of incompatible tissue is potentially disastrous. Ironically, patients with group O blood – the so-called universal donors – invariably face the longest wait for a new kidney because they are only compatible with others of the same blood group. People with blood belonging to groups A, B or AB are compatible with two or more groups in the ABO system.

Sometimes it is possible to vary the rules of ABO compatibility – for example, to give those in blood group B, which is only found in 8 per cent of the population, quicker access to transplantation. This is highly significant for many patients from ethnic minority groups, who are more likely to develop kidney failure and more likely to be in blood group B. Otherwise, these patients may linger for years on transplant waiting lists.

Tissue typing is the identification of cell surface markers, called antigens, which trigger rejection. These antigens are determined by a set of genes (human leucocyte antigen, HLA) passed on by parents to their children. They enable the immune system to recognise a graft as 'foreign'. The closer the HLA match of a recipient with the donor, the less likelihood there is of rejection. This is why acute rejection does not occur when a kidney is donated by an identical twin.

Once a patient is accepted onto the waiting list for a transplant, their details – name, blood group, HLA profile – are forwarded to the NHSBT centre in Bristol. Here, they are entered into a computerised registry of waiting recipients, which is scanned each time an organ becomes available for what is considered to be an 'optimum' or 'beneficial' match.

The third compatibility test – crossmatching – is performed once a kidney becomes available. By now the potential recipient has been called in to the transplant centre. Here, as part of the pre-transplant screening procedure, their serum is mixed in culture with lymphocytes (white blood cells) from the donor spleen or lymph nodes to see whether any cytotoxic (cell-destroying) antibodies are produced. Antibodies, protein molecules which attack foreign antigens, are the basic units of immunity. If they are seen in quantity when tissues from two different individuals are brought together, the crossmatch is said to be positive; in other words, the tissues are incompatible. If a transplant were to go ahead in the face of a positive crossmatch, hyper-acute rejection would set in immediately, causing rapid and unstoppable rejection of the graft.

One strategy enabling ABO-incompatible transplantation is proving particularly helpful for some renal patients who have would-be donors standing by. If the patient's level of antibodies to their intended donor is not too high, they are given a first infusion of the immunosuppressive drug rituximab a month before the transplant to suppress antibody production. A further infusion is given – in addition to other anti-rejection drugs – at the time of surgery.

The second arm of this technique, which has been developed in Sweden, the US and Japan, is a procedure called plasma exchange. This involves removal of the plasma, which is the colourless fluid component of the blood containing the antibodies, and replacing it with fresh plasma. This three-hour procedure is first performed ten days before the transplant and then on alternate days until the second post-operative day.

UK centres offering this mode of ABO-incompatible transplantation warn that the risks are slightly higher than for a good match transplant. They include loss of the graft owing to immediate rejection and a greater incidence of complications, such as infection or tumours arising from stronger doses of immunosuppression. However, the estimate is that around 70 per cent of such transplants would be functioning after the first year. This compares with a one-year graft survival of up to 96 per cent for conventionally matched grafts.

Another method involves the use of a technique known as antigen-specific immunoadsorption, also first introduced in Sweden and first used in the UK in 2005. Here again the would-be recipient is pretreated with rituximab and then attends four sessions during which his or her blood is passed through a column designed to filter out the antibodies which would cause rejection, leaving other, non-threatening antibodies unharmed. Experience up to now has shown that, once the kidney transplant has taken place, the level of unwanted antibodies remains suppressed.

Many kidney patients have a high level of preformed antibodies which have accumulated in response to immune-provoking events, such as repeated blood transfusions, previous failed transplants or multiple pregnancies. This makes it more difficult to find a beneficial match and means they will have longer to wait for a new kidney. Techniques are being developed to reduce the number of antibodies in these highly sensitised patients. Meanwhile, a mismatch is to be avoided not just because it threatens graft survival, but also because it provokes the production of even more of these antibodies, making it harder still to find a suitable kidney for re-transplant.

An ingenious tactic for overcoming incompatibility where there is a living donor in prospect is the paired-pooled donation system (see previous chapter), where would-be donor and recipient pairs are matched anonymously with other pairs in the same situation. In effect this means that prospective donor A is found to be compatible with waiting recipient Y, while Y's intended partner, donor Z, is matched up with waiting recipient B.

At the transplant hospital, while the six-hour crossmatching process is under way, the would-be recipient undergoes the usual battery of preparative investigations. Depending on the blood chemistry, they may also need to dialyse before being taken to theatre. Finally, if the results of all the tests are satisfactory and the crossmatch proves negative, the operation can go ahead. It is only on rare occasions that surgery has to be cancelled owing to last-minute findings, such as ECG changes suggesting a deterioration in heart condition or some hitherto undiagnosed infection.

Immunosuppressive protocols to fight rejection vary between transplant centres. Some give two anti-rejection drugs. Some rely on triple therapy – for instance, tacrolimus or ciclosporin and azathioprine or mycophenolate mofetil together with the steroid drug prednisolone. One or other of two monoclonal antibody preparations, basiliximab or daclizumab, are given intravenously immediately after the transplant. Kidney recipients may also be prescribed a range of drugs to counter some of the troublesome side-effects of the immunosuppressants (see Chapter 7). Typically they would receive antibiotics, antivirals and antifungals to combat infection – especially of the mouth – as well as various treatments to prevent stomach ulcers. There is also medication to prevent high blood pressure and raised cholesterol.

The operation itself, which takes about two to three hours, is the shortest and simplest of the organ transplant procedures. A long incision curves up from one or other bottom corners of the abdomen (usually on the right-hand side), exposing the site where the new kidney is to be inserted. The original artery and vein still attached to the donor kidney are anastomosed (joined) to vessels deep in the recipient's pelvic cavity. A rigid plastic tube known as a stent may be inserted into the donor ureter to prevent kinking or leakage and this will be left in place for about three months; the vessel is then anastomosed to the recipient's bladder. Except in rare cases, the person's own kidneys are left where they are.

The recipient leaves the operating theatre festooned with invasive equipment to assist post-operative care. The intravenous line and central venous catheter are removed within a day or two and the urinary catheter within two to five days. If the patient has previously been on peritoneal dialysis, the Tenckhoff catheter used for this will remain in place for several months – until the renal physician is satisfied that the new kidney is working well.

There are a number of surgical and other complications associated with kidney grafting, from wound infection – now very rare – to graft thrombosis. Often, these are hard to distinguish from the effects of acute rejection. Even so, excellent graft function is seen in almost all recipients of kidneys from live donors, as well as up to half of those receiving cadaveric kidneys, by the end of the first week. Of the rest, most are working within two to three weeks, although some grafted kidneys may take up to five to six weeks to begin producing urine.

When a transplanted kidney fails to work and there is no urine output it is often owing to the phenomenon known as acute tubular necrosis (ATN), a reversible shutdown attributable to the period of preservation. ATN mostly resolves within a week or two, but patients whose grafts are slow to pick up have to return temporarily to dialysis. This does not impede the recovery of the grafted kidney in any way.

While the twin spectres of infection and rejection continue to haunt the post-operative period, it is true to say that neither represents anywhere near the threat of earlier days. The risk from serious infection has fallen with the introduction of more refined immunosuppression in contrast to former regimens which more or less hammered the recipient's immune system into the ground.

Rejection is the process whereby donor tissue is recognised as foreign and destroyed by the recipient's immune system. There are two basic types: acute rejection, which occurs from one week to several months after surgery; and chronic rejection, a slow, long-term process resulting in gradual destruction of the graft. Acute rejection can usually be treated successfully with high-dose steroids; the effects of chronic rejection are irreversible.

These days rejection occurs in only about 20 per cent of cases within the first few weeks and most such episodes do not produce symptoms. Nevertheless, patients are briefed to watch out for early symptoms, such as pain or tenderness in the vicinity of the graft, fever, weight gain (from fluid retention) and decreased urine output. If there are no complications, kidney recipients are usually discharged from hospital after about ten days. However, there are still the clinic visits: two to three times a week for the first two months, then once weekly until the sixth month.

For patients who remain well, life gradually returns to normal and many claim that, once they are over the effects of surgery, they feel better than they have for years. It is often said that if a kidney graft is functioning well after three months it should continue to do so for some years. Regardless of the statistical averages, it is not uncommon to meet recipients with kidney grafts which have served them well for more than thirty years.

Chapter 7

Living With a New Organ

Solid organ transplants are performed either to save lives or to improve quality of life. People with terminal lung or liver failure would die without a transplant; those listed for heart transplant would otherwise die or be dependent on a machine. Kidney transplants free people from the tyranny of dialysis and, hopefully, lengthen their lives; dialysis patients are four times more likely to die than transplant recipients. Pancreas recipients no longer require daily insulin and are spared some of the serious long-term depredations of diabetes. Small bowel recipients are relieved of the misery and sometimes fatal complications of artificial feeding. In each case, transplantation offers the potential for a full and active life.

Kidney transplant is and will always remain the most successful and widely practised procedure, with 96 per cent of grafts from living donors and 93 per cent of cadaver organs functioning well at one year. With livers, hearts and lungs, the condition of patients referred for transplant varies greatly, from those who are up and about to others lying mortally ill in ICUs. Consequently, there can be considerable variation in survival rates. Figures quoted for one-year survival for these organs are respectively 91 per cent, 83 per cent and 79 per cent. The one-year success rate for pancreas transplants (72 per cent for pancreas only, 88 per cent for combined pancreas-kidney) refers to graft survival in that, just as the kidney recipient can return to dialysis, the patient whose pancreas fails can go back on insulin.

The honeymoon period may be rather stormy, of course, with one or two bouts of early (acute) rejection and endless clinic visits. An important objective of these early follow-up visits is to establish appropriate doses of the drugs used to prevent rejection. Successful immunosuppression is something of a juggling act between the need to prevent the immune system rejecting the new organ and yet not depressing it to such an extent that it can no longer fight infection. Acute rejection, occurring within the first few weeks of surgery, is now less common with the new generation of immunosuppressive drugs. It is usually treatable and only rarely causes graft failure. Chronic rejection – a slow, insidious process – remains a threat throughout the life of the transplanted organ, resulting in its gradual destruction.

The permutations of drugs used between transplant centres vary but, to forestall rejection, most regimens consist of triple therapy: either ciclosporin or tacrolimus together with azathioprine or mycophenolate mofetil (MMF) plus prednisolone (a steroid). Azathioprine was the first effective anti-rejection drug, introduced in 1962. It damps down the immune response by slowing production of immune cells. A newer alternative to azathioprine, mycophenolate mofetil is thought to reduce the likelihood of acute rejection, but it may carry higher overall risks than the older drug.

Ciclosporin, isolated from a soil fungus and brought into use from the early 1980s, was the first immunosuppressant to act specifically against the rejection process: it interrupts the cascade of events which take place in response to antibody from the grafted organ. Tacrolimus and sirolimus are two more recent alternatives to ciclosporin. Other new drugs include basiliximab and daclizumab, two monoclonal antibody preparations which may be used in combination with other drugs immediately post-transplant.

It is no secret that immunosuppressive drugs give rise to a long list of unwanted side-effects, ranging from excessive hair growth to kidney damage and tumour formation, including male breast cancer. Ciclosporin, for instance, is a powerful weapon in the armoury, but it is also highly nephrotoxic – harmful to the kidneys. By using it in low doses, combined with azathioprine or MMF, a good level of immunosuppression can be achieved with minimum risk to the kidneys. The addition of a steroid (prednisolone) minimises the toxic effects of these other drugs while maximising benefits, although long-term use of this drug is associated with osteoporosis (bone thinning). Ciclosporin, tacrolimus and prednisolone can all trigger diabetes. Following an initial high-dose bombardment for maybe the first fortnight following a transplant, doses of these powerful drugs can be lowered for maintenance treatment.

Like cancer patients, recipients whose immune systems have been knocked out by medication are at greatly increased risk of infection, especially from viruses that do not affect healthy people; in this sense they are said to be opportunistic. Cytomegalovirus (CMV), for instance, one of the herpes group of viruses, is widely present in the general population, where it is mostly harmless, but it can cause severe problems in transplant recipients. For this reason, antivirals are given to forestall CMV infection in patients thought to be at risk.

The risk from infection declines after the first three months but the threat of rejection continues. Chronic rejection is the commonest cause of graft failure, although, increasingly, loss of a transplanted organ is seen to be the final outcome of damage owing to several factors, some of which have nothing to do with immunity as such. Aside from acute rejection, they include: damage to the organ incurred before the transplant; viral infection; and the cumulative toxic effects of various anti-rejection drugs.

Typically, this downward spiral is seen in kidney and heart recipients, particularly in those who have had repeated episodes of acute rejection. There is a gradual loss of function in the grafted organ and, while the degenerative process may flatten out for a time, graft failure is inevitable. There is no specific treatment to stop this from happening. Curiously, this process of attrition is far less evident among liver recipients, of whom less than 5 per cent experience chronic rejection. The liver is thought to be immunologically privileged to some extent and, where more than one organ is transplanted, this protection embraces other grafts as well.

An answer to rejection, something which overshadows the lives of almost all organ recipients, is regarded as the holy grail of the transplant community. Curiously, specialists at the Westmead Children's Hospital in Sydney, Australia, believe they chanced upon something which could point the way in the case of teenager Demi-Lee Brennan. In 2001, after her liver had been wrecked by a viral hepatitis, 9-year-old Demi-Lee received the liver of a 12-year-old boy who had died following a brain injury. She was started on immunosuppressive medication and appeared to do well. Then, nine months later, she became critically ill again with a blood disorder, causing the red blood cells to break down. It was during investigation and treatment for this condition that it was found that, with her own immune system suppressed, Demi-Lee's O-negative blood had been replaced by blood from the donor's group (O-positive) and that somehow she had inherited his immune system – something hitherto unheard of in transplantation.

What seems to have happened was that stem cells in the donor liver had invaded Demi-Lee's bone marrow – the site of red blood cell production – overwhelming it, after which it began producing O-positive blood. She even had to be re-vaccinated against measles and mumps as the dead boy had not received these vaccinations. She was taken off all immunosuppressive drugs in the course of the second post-transplant year and has had no complications in the years since. Medical scientists believe that scrutiny of the Demi-Lee phenomenon – described by one doctor as a 'one in six billion miracle' – may open the way to solving the problem of rejection.

While the Australian case is unique, US transplant teams have had some success in grafting donor immune cells into organ recipients in order to 'kid' their immune systems into recognising donor organs as their own. This engineered tolerance has enabled some patients' anti-rejection drugs to be withdrawn. Another strategy which has been taken up by some transplant centres is the use of a monoclonal antibody (alemtuzumab) as induction therapy at the time of transplant. This has the effect of depleting the recipient's white blood cells, which are important in immunity, and enabling use of much lower dosages of anti-rejection drugs. With the new organ in place, lymphocyte production is allowed to resume over a period of time.

Researchers in Britain and the US are focusing on a distinct pattern of gene expression which has been identified in kidney recipients who, for whatever reason, have stopped taking their immunosuppressive medication but who have not experienced rejection. This work could indicate which organ recipients could reduce or discontinue their immunotherapy without risk of incurring rejection.

Less frequent than rejection but still a threat to graft survival is the recurrence of the original disease. This is a particular risk in patients with some of the genetic or metabolic diseases seen in transplant centres. Nobody knows to what extent recurrence goes on, since it is often presumed to be chronic rejection. However, reappearance of the old disease does not automatically imply loss of the graft. Often, the condition remains 'silent' and may only be discovered by chance when a biopsy is taken.

Also of concern is the association of immunosuppression with certain cancers. In fact, for organ recipients the risk of malignancy is about three times as high as it is for the UK population in general. Transplant patients do not suffer a higher incidence of the common cancers, but they are at greatly increased risk of some more unusual forms, such as various lymphomas (cancer of the lymph nodes), Kaposi's sarcoma (a malignant tumour arising from blood vessels within the skin) and skin cancers; women recipients are also at greater risk of genital cancers. A heightened risk of skin cancer means that transplant recipients must cover up in strong sunshine. High rates of cancer are attributed not so much to any one drug as to the overall potency of immunosuppressive therapy. However, there is one anti-rejection drug – sirolimus – which has been seen to eradicate Kaposi's sarcoma.

In the long term, inevitably, those respectable one-year survival figures begin to fall away. Take kidney recipients, for instance. Less than 20 per cent will have suffered acute rejection in the first three months post-transplant but, as time goes on, hypertension can be a problem and one in twenty of them – especially those of black or South Asian origin – will develop permanent diabetes requiring insulin treatment. About 30 per cent of kidney recipients develop an eminently curable skin cancer after ten years of immunosuppression. However, by far the majority do very well.

The average lifespan of a transplanted kidney is ten years if it came from a cadaver donor, about twelve years for one from a living related donor and something in between these two figures in the case of living unrelated donation. More often than not, when a grafted kidney fails it has to be removed. This operation, usually performed through the old incision, can be technically more demanding than the original transplant owing to inflammation and the scarring caused by rejection. Even so, many patients opt for a further transplant. Kept going on dialysis, they may face a longer wait for a new kidney the second time around.

The fate of second and subsequent grafts depends on what happened with the original transplant. If it was lost to early rejection, the outlook is not so good. But where a kidney has lasted for more than a year, or has failed earlier for reasons other than rejection, the prognosis is brighter. Overall, graft survival rates after second attempts are 10–15 per cent lower than for primary transplants. It is not uncommon to meet people who have had several kidney transplants.

People with severe unstable diabetes sometimes undergo pancreas-only transplant, although a simultaneous pancreas-kidney (SPK) graft is more common. One-year graft survival rates are 72 per cent for pancreas only and 88 per cent for SPK. A new pancreas makes for better survival than chronic insulin treatment, probably because it curbs long-term diabetic problems. Although diabetic patients replace insulin dependence with a lifetime requirement for immunosuppressive therapy, most find that they have fewer dietary and other restrictions and a better quality of life.

It is always said that when someone does well after a liver transplant, they do very well; when they do badly, the clinical course may be frankly terrible. For a minority of liver recipients the post-transplant course is strewn with serious complications, sometimes resulting in lengthy spells in hospital. Between 10 and 20 per cent of grafted livers fail, often within the first month. There are many reasons for this early fallout, including the fact that some donor livers simply do not commence functioning. In this case the patient may be offered a swift re-transplant; here, too, survival rates are lower.

Inevitably, some very sick recipients do not survive. Of those dying in the first year, most do so within the first sixty days. Sepsis and multi-organ failure are responsible for more than half of all these deaths. Again, this nightmare scenario only affects a minority. After five years more than three quarters of liver recipients are still alive; survival at fifteen years is 58 per cent. Statisticians have calculated that the average life expectancy of an adult liver transplant recipient is twenty-two years.

Considering one in three heart transplant recipients will have been too ill to leave hospital in the run-up to surgery, the success of this transplant – currently quoted as 83 per cent survival at one year – is impressive. The most common cause of early death, occurring in 5 to 10 per cent of heart recipients, is failure of the graft to function. The risk of death increases if the new heart is implanted more than three hours after removal from the donor, although this problem should be eased with the introduction of organ preservation equipment incorporating continuous blood flow.

In general, heart recipients who survive the first year tend to do well; although their exercise tolerance is more limited than that of healthy individuals. This may be partly owing to the fact that there is no nerve supply to the transplanted heart (although the nerve supply has been seen to regenerate after some years). At five years, one third of recipients have coronary artery disease (the most common cause of late death after a heart transplant); one third have abnormal kidney function; and one fifth will have had a cancer of some kind. For some reason, heart recipients are twice as likely to develop skin cancer as kidney recipients; almost half go on to get skin cancer – although few actually die from it – within fifteen years. The twenty-year survival rate following heart transplantation is 15 per cent.

Lung transplant success rates trail somewhat behind those of the other procedures, with 79 per cent survival at one year and 56 per cent at five years. Rates of infection are higher than in other solid organ populations, especially in the first six months. Early deaths are the result of either this or poor graft function. Chronic rejection can arise as early as six months post-transplant, when the small airways become narrowed by scar tissue, a condition known as obliterative bronchiolitis. Re-transplantation of lungs is rare because it poses much higher risks than a primary transplant.

Women who have had lung transplants are thought to be more vulnerable than other organ recipients to complications arising from pregnancy. In their case there is an increased risk of rejection if pregnancy ensues within two to three years of a transplant. All women transplant recipients are urged to avoid pregnancy for at least a year and the evidence is that most of those becoming pregnant – mostly kidney recipients – are rewarded with live births. A Hertfordshire woman made history recently by becoming the first double organ recipient (pancreas and kidney) to become a mother.

A somewhat unnerving finding, reported in 2002, is that recipients receiving organs from female donors are more likely to reject than those grafted with organs donated by men. This came out when researchers at the University of Heidelberg analysed a worldwide database of more than 124,000 kidney transplants, 25,000 heart transplants and 16,000 liver transplants. They found that the risk of a male recipient losing a kidney was 22 per cent higher when the donor was a woman. Women were at 15 per cent greater risk of losing the kidney if the donor was a woman. Both sexes were at slightly increased risk of dying after receiving organs from female donors.

A Swiss-led study, carried out six years later in collaboration with the Heidelberg group, reported on data from 195,156 kidney transplants carried out across Europe between 1985 and 2004. They found that men have a much better survival rate with male kidneys but females are not harmed by receiving a male kidney. They concluded that male kidneys contain more nephrons (the kidneys' active units of excretion) than female ones, which makes them more robust. Why these discrepancies occur is not known, although one theory is that women mount a much stronger immune response than men. At the time this later report appeared, UK Transplant, as it then was, insisted its own survey had found no difference in rejection rates.

A more recent finding is that heart transplant patients are more likely to survive if they receive an organ from a donor of the same sex. A study of more than 18,000 heart recipients, conducted by researchers at Johns Hopkins University in Baltimore, found that death rates rose by a fifth where female patients had received men's hearts. The study also showed that gender-matched transplants yielded a 25 per cent decline in the thirty-day death rate and a 20 per cent lower one-year death rate; lower rates of rejection were apparent in the long term. Here again, why this should be so is not clear in that male and female hearts are identical except for size. Realistically, gender matching is hardly feasible in the UK, where at the moment less than 200 heart transplants are being performed each year.

Organ recipients often find it takes longer to come to terms psychologically with a transplant than to adjust to changed physical circumstances. They experience a range of emotions, sometimes compounded by the effects of the powerful drugs they are taking. It is well known that a significant number of heart recipients, for instance, conceal feelings of distress which are quite at odds with their apparent well-being. Many organ recipients have strong feelings about the donor, although not all of them can cope with writing to the donor family. Some, weathering patches of post-transplant depression, experience what might almost be classed as survivor guilt. One heart-lung recipient says: 'You'll be going along fine and then one day it hits you between the eyes – that someone has had to die to give you this new life.'

Fortunately, despite all the setbacks and the sheer stress of undergoing a transplant, the majority of recipients enjoy years of post-transplant life relatively free of complications. The only cloud on their horizon, given that no graft is immortal, is how long their new organ will last. This question is, of course, unanswerable, since transplanted organs have been known to function for anything from a few hours to several decades. However, there have been some remarkable survivals. The world's longest-living heart recipient was a businessman in Ohio, Tony Huesman, who survived thirty-one years on a single donated organ. Transplanted in 1978 for disease of the heart muscle known as cardiomyopathy, he died of an aggressive skin cancer (melanoma) in August 2009, aged 51. Britain's longest-surviving heart recipient, 78-year-old Joe Burnside, died in October 2008, some twenty-eight years after receiving his new heart. A number of liver and kidney recipients have survived more than two decades on a single graft.

Chapter 8

Some Way in the Future

It has to be said that there will never be enough organs available for transplantation. Even if the entire adult population of the UK were to sign up to the ODR there still wouldn't be enough. For one thing, most people do not die in circumstances appropriate to donation. Also, of course, many of the organs that are offered for donation are frankly unusable. Meanwhile, the waiting lists for organs are only the tip of the iceberg. Most of the conditions for which transplantation is the treatment of choice are on the increase and, because of the organ shortfall, only a small percentage of patients are referred to transplant centres. It is this scarcity of organs that is driving the quest for alternatives to transplantation.

Currently there are three broad avenues of research: xenotransplantation, using organs from animals; various kinds of cell therapy; and the use of artificial organs. Of these, xenotransplantation has the longest and most colourful record, dating back more than a century to a time when human donation would not have been countenanced. Since these early attempts were spectacularly unsuccessful, interest in xenotransplantation waned. It revived briefly in the 1960s, when a number of xenografts were attempted; none of the adult recipients survived more than a few days. The most notorious attempt at xenografting, the Baby Fae case in California, occurred in 1984, when a baby girl was given the heart of a baboon; she survived for twenty days. In all cases the problem was that the human immune system attacks tissues from other species far more aggressively than it does tissues from incompatible human beings.

As time went on there was a move away from using organs from non-human primates since there was a high risk of viral transmission and, in any case, some species were on the endangered list. Also, of course, to many people it was morally repugnant to make use of primates – close relatives of ours – in this way. Attention turned to pigs as being phylogenetically more distant from the human race. The attributes which commend the use of pigs in this context are that they are more prolific than primates, producing large litters at frequent intervals, and their organs are anatomically similar to our own.

First, there was a huge immunological barrier to be overcome. Human beings possess pre-formed antibodies to antigens present in non-primate species, including pigs. If a pig organ is transplanted into a human being, the person's immune system mounts a swift and powerful reaction, sometimes causing the organ to fail within minutes. Consequently, a great deal of research effort has been directed towards tinkering with pigs' genes to produce transgenic specimens whose organs would be less inimical to the human immune system.

Then there is the risk of introducing infectious agents from animals to human beings. The threat from many disease pathogens could be kept at bay by rearing genetically modified pigs in tightly controlled colonies. However, this would be no protection against the inadvertent transmission of viruses. Workers in the field were dismayed, for example, by the discovery in the late 1990s that pig cells could transmit porcine endogenous viruses (PERVs) to human cells in the laboratory. The fear is that the dormant viral DNA present in the pig genome could become active in a transplanted organ.

However, when samples were taken from people who had been treated with various pig tissues – heart valves, neuronal cells for Parkinson's – over some years no evidence of transmission was found. While pigs have been genetically modified to counter PERVs, it does mean that, if pig organs were to be used for human transplants, both the recipients and their families would face lifelong monitoring for evidence of viral transmission.

People with diabetes may well be the first to benefit from genetically modified pigs' tissues. Already a company in New Zealand is undertaking human trials using cells coated in alginate, a substance extracted from seaweed, which should prevent the human immune system from recognising them as 'foreign'. The cells are implanted into the patient's abdomen, from where they begin to produce insulin.

Advocates of xenotransplantation point to a long list of benefits which would ensue from the use of animal organs:

- many more lives would be saved;
- there would be no further need to acquire organs from human beings (either living or dead);
- the organs used for grafting would be of optimum quality;
- it would be possible to offer transplants to older people who normally are not accepted onto waiting lists today;
- immunosuppression could be reduced or perhaps even eliminated altogether;
- there would be huge cost savings to be made from the much reduced need for dialysis and for the intensive care of patients in terminal organ failure.

Whether their enthusiasm will be shared by the public remains to be seen. In 2004, a Wellcome Trust survey showed that the British public had severe reservations about xenotransplantation. There was fierce criticism of the use of genetically modified animals to populate 'organs farms'. Possibly more acceptable would be a hybrid creation using a mixture of porcine and human tissue. One idea is to strip down an animal heart, using a chemical to dissolve away the flesh so that only the basic collagen framework remains. This framework is then seeded with tissue grown from human stem cells. This assembly sidesteps the rejection issue altogether. Collagen, the principal constituent of fibrous connective tissue, is said to be 'immunologically inert' and the cells would come either from the intended recipient or from someone whose tissues are compatible.

More groups are now turning to this technique, a combination of xenotransplantation and stem-cell science, to create experimental muscle and livers as well as hearts. Of course, human organs could also be used for this purpose, perhaps some of those which are not suitable for grafting in their entirety or some which cannot be accessed within the normal timescale for transplantation.

This kind of tissue engineering has already been used to create replacement airways. First to benefit, in Barcelona in 2008, was a 30-year-old Colombian woman whose trachea had been damaged by tuberculosis. She received a partial graft developed from a de-cellularised windpipe from a cadaver donor and stem cells taken from her own bone marrow. In Britain, the first recipient of a tissue-engineered trachea was a 10-year-old boy who had been born without an adequate windpipe. His transplant – a nine-hour procedure – took place at Great Ormond Street Hospital in March 2010.

Stem cells are cells which as yet have not assumed a role in life: they are undifferentiated. This is in contrast to differentiated cells – those which have become specialised as contributing to any one of the human body's 200 tissues. An embryonic stem cell is formed when a sperm cell fertilises an egg cell (ovum), forming a one-cell embryo. The human organism develops from this one totipotent cell. After a few days this single cell will have multiplied to form a blastocyst, and it is from this minuscule structure that human embryonic stem cells (hESCs) are taken for research. The problem here is an ethical one: the fact that at present the acquisition of stem cells destroys the embryo. In the UK, scientists can only use human embryos for research for up to fourteen days after fertilisation.

Here again, diabetic patients may be among the first to benefit, with at least two US biotech firms turning hESCs into insulin-producing cells. Similarly, pioneers in a number of centres are seeking to use heart muscle cells derived from hESCs to treat patients whose hearts have been damaged. In 2005, researchers from London's Imperial College reported success in manipulating hESCs to convert into lung cells. The team, led by the distinguished scientist Professor Dame Julia Polak – herself a heart-lung recipient – saw this as a major step towards being able to repair diseased lung tissue or to build human lungs for transplantation.

The following year came news of the first bio-artificial liver, developed by a team from Newcastle University. The miniature organ, about the size of a one-penny piece, was built from stem cells derived from umbilical cord blood – a source thought to be ethically more acceptable than the actual embryo. This tiny prototype, already used for drug testing, is seen as a major step in creating a full-sized liver. Several other groups are working on both artificial and bio-artificial livers, but so far there has been limited success in replicating this immensely versatile organ.

Meanwhile, the paediatric liver service at King's College Hospital in south London has been using injections of hepatocytes – the functional cells of the liver – to treat children with inherited liver disease. Healthy liver cells, taken from donated organs, are injected into the portal vein, which conveys nutrient-rich blood from the intestines to the liver. These donor cells colonise the liver, supplementing the child's own hepatocytes. Because of the shortage of donated liver tissue, King's researchers are collaborating with other groups to develop ways of getting human hepatocytes to proliferate in the laboratory. While the procedure is not likely to replace transplantation of the whole organ for adults with terminal liver failure, if hepatocytes can be made available in sufficient quantity this strategy could be of use for adult patients with less advanced disease or, in certain cases, as a bridge to transplantation.

Because of the controversy surrounding embryonic stem cells, researchers are exploring other sources of stem cells. Adult stem cells are found in various sites in the body, in particular the bone marrow. The function of adult stem cells is to replenish cells lost by damage or depletion. Already partly specialised, adult stem cells are harder to find than embryonic ones and do not possess the same potential. However, they have been reprogrammed in the laboratory to differentiate into cell types with more potential (induced pluripotent stem cells). The great value of adult stem cells is that any future therapy could make use of the patient's own stem cells, or those from a compatible human donor, so as to minimise the chance of rejection.

Given the shortage of donor hearts, stem cells could have a major role to play in easing the burden of heart failure. Recent research has focused on developing tissue-engineered material to regenerate damaged heart muscle. What is believed to be the first whole organ created in a laboratory was reported in 2008, when a team at the University of Minnesota rebuilt a rat's heart. Here again, the technique was to dissolve away the muscle of a dead rat's heart, leaving a scaffolding of connective tissue which was then reclothed with stem cells from younger rats. After a few days in culture, the cells set up a rhythmic beat and, later still, the rebuilt organ began to pump blood – to the astonishment of the research team.

Outside the laboratory a recent innovation is combination therapy – saving a dying patient by fitting an artificial heart and at the same time injecting stem cells in a bid to rebuild the failed heart. This procedure – believed to be the first of its kind in the world – was pioneered by a British cardiothoracic surgeon in 2009 on a Greek patient in Thessalonika, since as yet there is no funding for it in this country. The surgeon's estimate is that some 12,000 patients a year in the UK could benefit from the combined procedure.

Most of the so-called artificial hearts are in fact ventricular assist devices (VADs) as distinct from true artificial hearts which take over the complete function of patients' hearts. VADs are made to assist either the right ventricle (RVADs) or the left ventricle (LVADs) and the latter are much the most commonly used. Most of the older VADs did not live up to expectations. They either proved inadequate for the task or, more often, set up unwanted side-effects like blood clots or infection. These devices were mostly seen as providing a bridge to transplantation, although some have been associated with survival for several years. Britain's longest survivor was Peter Houghton, a former social worker turned psychotherapist, who had been fitted with a Jarvik 2000 heart pump at Oxford's John Radcliffe Infirmary in June 2000. He died in November 2007, having written one book and co-authored another, fund-raised and travelled the world to publicise the Radcliffe's artificial heart programme.

There have been instances where use of an LVAD has taken the strain, as it were, allowing the native heart to heal. A leading British transplant centre, Harefield Hospital in Uxbridge, Middlesex, ran a trial (the Harefield Recovery Protocol Study, HARPS, reported in 2006), to establish whether combining use of LVADs and drugs would enable the heart to recover 'to a point where it could work effectively without assistance and without a recurrence of heart failure'. Frequent monitoring showed significant improvement in patients entered in the trial and, once 'satisfactory heart function' could be shown for fifteen minutes with the LVADs switched off, the devices were removed. Roughly three quarters of patients who received the full course of combination therapy recovered; of these, 88.9 per cent had not suffered a recurrence after five years. These patients were spared transplantation and were able to enjoy greatly improved quality of life.

With results as compelling as those from HARPS, it is possible that these devices may ultimately come to replace heart transplantation.

The idea of a permanent implantable pump is increasingly attractive to heart specialists. Among the new generation of devices is the Australian-made HeartWare pump which, battery-driven and small enough to lodge in the sac surrounding the heart, is already available in the UK. However, a number of centres continue to strive for the perfect artificial heart. There are a couple of prototype contenders in the US and a French team, led by Professor Alain Carpentier, has claimed that its prototype, a fully implantable artificial heart, will be ready for clinical trials some time in 2011. Said to beat like the real thing, it is being developed jointly by start-up company Carmat and EADS, the European aerospace giant responsible for the Airbus. The French model has already been tested successfully in animals.

It is perhaps not surprising that Wilhelm Kolff, the Dutch physician who invented the first artificial kidney, is said to have spent his declining years modelling a new heart pump. Kolff's 'rotating drum', developed in occupied Holland during World War II, became the forerunner of later dialysis machines. A born inventor, after moving to the US in 1950, Kolff played a leading role in a number of major innovations, including the heart-lung machine (1955) and the world's first permanent artificial heart, the Jarvik-7, which, with its 180 kg (400 lb) air compressor, was first used in 1982 in a bid to save a retired Seattle dentist, 61-year-old Barney Clark. Dr Clark, who had been within hours of death from congestive heart failure, survived in the full glare of global publicity for a further, troubled 112 days.

By the time of Wilhelm Kolff's death, aged 98, in Pennsylvania in 2009, there were already several wearable dialysis devices in development. Prominent among these was a Californian model, the automated wearable artificial kidney (AWAK), which weighed 2.7 kg (6 lb) at its unveiling in late 2009 but which its developers hope to reduce to 0.9 kg (2 lb) by the time it comes to market. The AWAK will enable 'dialysis-on-the-go', according to its inventors, freeing patients in renal failure from the 'servitude' of conventional dialysis.

Also in development are implantable dialysis devices, notably a collaborative one involving scientists from the Cleveland Clinic, the University of California at San Francisco and the University of Michigan in Ann Arbor. The planned device is a hybrid, consisting of high-tech nanoscale silicon membranes and living kidney cells. It is designed to free users from having to use not only machinery but also dialysate fluid.

Elsewhere, just as with the other organs, there are schemes going ahead for an artificial pancreas. In spring 2010 it was announced that researchers from Massachusetts General Hospital, in collaboration with biomedical engineers from the University of Boston, had produced a prototype which monitors and regulates blood-sugar levels. Intended for people with Type 1 diabetes, the artificial endocrine pancreas is in effect a double pump, dispensing insulin and, when necessary, automatically secreting glucagon, a hormone which draws on glucose reserves in the liver, raising blood-sugar levels if they go too low so as to forestall hypoglycaemia. The next step in the programme is to reduce the computerised device to a portable system about the size of a mobile phone.

Specialists at the same hospital had caused a stir two years earlier with their account of an experiment to blitz the immune system so that organs can be transplanted without the need for immunosuppressants. At Massachusetts General Hospital five kidney recipients received pretreatment with chemotherapy, radiation and steroids, targeting the bone marrow so that the white blood cells which attack a donor organ (T-cells) would be obliterated. Post-operatively they were given intravenous infusions of cells from their donors' bone marrow. The idea was that, as the patients' own weakened systems recovered, the donor bone marrow would generate new T-cells, creating in effect a hybrid immune system. By the time the Boston clinicians' report appeared, in January 2008, four of the five treated recipients had been free of immunosuppressive therapy for more than five years. This is a particularly significant outcome, because the kidney recipients had not been closely matched with their donors, which means the chances of rejection would have been higher than they would following a closely matched transaction.

At the same time a group from Stanford University in Palo Alto, California, reported a similar attempt but with perfectly matched donors and a slightly less robust attack on the immune system. There were six kidney recipients who featured in the experiment, one of whom had not required immunosuppressive drugs for more than two years.

These attempts to manipulate the immune system are reminiscent of the remarkable story of the 9-year-old Australian liver recipient Demi-Lee (see Chapter 7), where the desired outcome somehow occurred naturally. It was only when Demi-Lee became seriously ill ten months after her transplant in 2001 that tests revealed that she had acquired both the immune system and the blood group of her donor. Her experience, regarded as nothing short of a miracle at the time, has no doubt inspired some of the subsequent experimental work.

Nobody seems to know why the induced immune tolerance reported from Boston and Stanford works. It is possible that the pretreatment these investigators used prevents the recipient's own T-cells from mounting a response to donated tissue. For recipients the choice would be between an initial intensive bombardment or the prospect of spending the rest of their lives on immunosuppressive drugs with all the heightened risk of infection, kidney damage and certain cancers. However, induced tolerance is unlikely to become generally available any time soon, not least because the time lag between bombardment of the native T-cells, which play a key role in fighting infection, and the maturation of the hybrid immune system would leave recipients open to all manner of pathogens.

The most striking development in this area is a new drug, announced in September 2010, which could increase the 'shelf life' of donated organs and, too, extend the life of grafts. The new drug, engineered at King's College in London, is a synthetic concoction of the protein molecules which, in life, are present on the surface of organs to act as a restraint on the immune system. However, these molecules are lost when the organ is retrieved from the donor and the blood supply ceases. The experimental drug, called mirococept, would be infused into the donor organ to combat damage during transit and after transplant surgery. If trials are successful, the treatment could go a long way to reducing wastage of organs and also allow a reduction in dosages of immunosuppressants. The King's College researchers believe the drug could be made available to hospitals within five years.

As the clamour for new organs intensifies, so developments on the periphery of transplantation come to increasing prominence. The attraction of the new technologies is not least that they hold out the hope of circumventing the whole problem of organ rejection. But it is true to say that all three of the alternatives to conventional grafting –

xenotransplantation, stem cell regeneration and artificial organs – are still some way in the future. For the time being the quest for tolerance, for being able to dispense altogether with immunosuppressive drugs, remains the holy grail of the transplant community.

Selected Case Histories

Deborah's Story

A Charmed Life

A born entrepreneur, Deborah Duval has managed to make time for no less than three organ transplants in a colourful career which has ranged all the way from showbiz to cross-country running, charity work, NHS committees and public speaking. She is perhaps best known as editor of the National Kidney Federation's official quarterly *Kidney Life*, which serves a readership of more than 25,000, and, too, as an impassioned champion of kidney patients' rights.

Deborah's kidneys failed as a late consequence of the diabetes she had developed as an 11-year-old in Cornwall. First, living in London in her twenties, she began to experience other diabetic complications, including peripheral nerve problems and eye disease. Then, after marrying and trying unsuccessfully for two years for a baby, she was told of the kidney damage when she went for gynaecological investigation back near her home in Cornwall.

The deterioration continued for more than three years until, in February 1993, Deborah started peritoneal dialysis. 'I chose this method because I was in a stable marriage where I believed this change in my appearance would not matter. I had not taken into consideration the huge impact it would have on my perception of myself and in turn the effect it would have on my personality.' So began a nightmare round of vomiting, tiredness and anaemia. 'In my marriage I grew to detest the plastic PD catheter dangling from my stomach, and this, combined with a particularly nasty renal itch, night-time cramps and general all-over lethargy meant bedtime was a problem for me.'

Within a few months Deborah had become a shadow of her former self. However, meanwhile she had discovered, and researched, the possibility of a pancreas-kidney transplant and so the Cornwall consultant referred her to the Royal Liverpool University Hospital for investigations. In October 1994 she underwent the combined transplant. After a few blips, including further spells in surgery and a brief episode of rejection, she went home just before Christmas.

But things were not the same. 'My husband went to great lengths to make me as comfortable as possible but he clearly mourned the loss of the woman he had married ... Our relationship had changed. The years of dealing with several chronic conditions had become the focus of our life together almost to the exclusion of anything else. My illness had become bigger than us. So we parted, but on good terms.'

Soon after the marriage broke up the transplanted kidney failed and by February 1998 Deborah was back on dialysis – haemodialysis this time since 'It suited my life much better.' Later that year she moved from Cornwall to Hampshire and came under the care of a Portsmouth hospital. But here the local purchasing authority would only fund two dialysis sessions per week, so by special arrangement she found herself driving back to the Treliske Hospital in Truro once a week for an essential third session. It was this experience which later prompted her to serve on an NHS south-west regional committee responsible for ensuring optimum treatment for patients in renal failure. 'During my time here the practice of under-dialysing renal patients was outlawed nationally – something for which I'd been campaigning for years.'

After just over a year on haemodialysis Deborah went back to the Liverpool hospital in May 1999 for a further kidney transplant – the second of the 'three most precious gifts in my life'. The new kidney worked well and Deborah continued expanding the company which she had set up five years earlier, organising villa holidays in Florida. She also continued speaking at renal courses to give nurses and junior medical staff some insight into the impact of chronic renal disease.

But then, three years after the kidney transplant, rejection knocked out the grafted pancreas. By now living in Buckinghamshire with her new partner, Geoff, Deborah went back on the waiting list. A new pancreas became available in February 2008 and the operation took place at the Churchill Hospital in Oxford. Again, the transplant went well and within a few months Deborah was developing a whole new business, this time in lingerie, catering in particular for women with special needs, such as accident victims and mastectomy patients.

Still kept busy with writing – including a book on women's experiences of renal disease – and with speaking engagements both in the UK and overseas, Deborah has learned to roll with the punches. 'I suppose I've had my ups and downs,' she says, 'but I do honestly consider that I lead a charmed life.'

Ernesto's Story

Less Than a 5 Per Cent Chance

When they took Ernesto Antonio into theatre for a heart transplant, they gave him less than a 5 per cent chance of survival. After nearly three months in a hospital bed, unable to care for himself or keep down food, the chances were slim. 'There was no muscle left on him,' says his wife, Kate. 'He looked like a Belsen victim. I don't know how he got through it. He must have had something else going for him apart from all the nursing care and surgical skill ...'

Ernesto was born and raised in Ireland. Until the summer of 1999 he'd been a fit, healthy young man. True, he'd had rheumatic fever when he was eighteen but he'd got over that, completed his training as a nurse at Galway University Hospital and, in his spare time, was a keen sportsman. Only a year previously he'd cycled across the Middle East for charity – '500 miles across the desert' – in memory of a friend who had died of leukaemia. Kate and he had met as theatre nurses at Oldchurch Hospital, Romford, Essex, eleven years previously and were enjoying their work and caring for their 5-year-old daughter, Isabella.

Then in May, still only thirty-five, Ernesto developed a chest infection. Despite courses of antibiotics, he found he was becoming increasingly breathless and exhausted. Being a nurse, he'd begun to suspect what the trouble was and several times asked his doctor for an 'echo' – echocardiography, which is an examination using ultrasound to investigate the action of the heart. But instead the doctor insisted it was asthma and prescribed inhalers. Next, when a chest X-ray showed a massively enlarged heart, he told Ernesto it was because he did so much cycling. Finally, he agreed to send him for an echo when he came back from holiday in Ireland.

Arriving in Galway on 6 August 1999, Ernesto was almost too tired to stand up and within four days he was admitted to the hospital where he'd trained. Here, too, they thought at first it was asthma, but when they checked his lung function and watched his legs blow up like balloons, they realised it was heart failure and sent him to the coronary care unit. His condition continued to deteriorate and when his liver and kidneys began to fail he was moved to intensive care. After three weeks the decision was taken to transfer him to the Mater Misericordiae Hospital in Dublin. Here he was swiftly listed for transplant.

By now critically ill, Ernesto had two 'bad calls', as they are known. 'I was all prepped and ready,' he says, 'and then the first heart that came up was too small. The second time the surgeon told me that when he got to the referring hospital the donor heart was almost in as bad shape as my own.' A third heart became available on the very day (26 October) that the family was warned that the end was near. Kate, who had been nursing Ernesto herself, recalls: 'The surgeon had just come back after assessing the donor heart and as he came down the corridor he gave me the thumbs up.'

Ernesto said: 'I was very lucky that the surgeons at the Mater had the courage to transplant me as I was so ill. Many surgeons would not even have considered it. In the end the staff at the hospital were calling me Lazarus or the Miracle Man.'

Ernesto came out of surgery alive – but barely. He knew nothing for a further three weeks as he fought off repeated infections. A tracheotomy was carried out to aid his respiratory effort and wean him from the ventilator which was keeping him alive. Then came a real landmark on the road to recovery: the day, towards the end of November, when he could be weaned off the ventilator completely. He was transferred to a high-dependency unit on 22 December and there, on Christmas Eve, he stood up and took his first step in five months. On Christmas Day, removal of the nasogastric tube through which he had been fed since August heralded a return to normality.

Ernesto was discharged from hospital in February 2000. He was still only little more than half the weight he'd been before he became ill. Progress was slow but fairly steady. By August he was able to start back at work part time and he resumed full-time nursing a year later, although, he says, 'It took five years to get my full strength back.'

Even so, Ernesto was impatient to show what a heart recipient could achieve – largely as a means of promoting organ donation. With this in mind, he embarked on a gruelling schedule of sports training, leaving the house at 6.00 a.m. to run or cycle for an hour before going to work.

On 31 December 2003, his fortieth birthday, he signed up for the London Triathlon. He completed his first half marathon in April 2005 and, 'in a moment of madness', entered the Dublin City Marathon. There, he ran past the hospital which had saved his life and now brought back so many memories. In 2006, he and two other organ recipients got together as the first ever team of its kind to take part in the London Triathlon. He cycled 40 km in one hour and fifteen minutes.

Ernesto's next success, two months after swimming the Bay of Galway in July 2010, was the fulfilling of a long-held ambition: the ascent of Mount Kilimanjaro. Having searched the Internet for information on heart transplants and altitude sickness, he linked up with a group at Heathrow and set off for East Africa. Over the next few days the group trekked upwards through rainforest, moorland and high, chill desert before the summit zone of Africa's highest mountain.

At 3,000 m, Ernesto was troubled by the thumping headache which is common at high altitude. On day three (4,000 m) he was soon battling altitude sickness. Wretchedly cold, nauseous and fatigued, he struggled on. 'Tears rolled down my face, hidden by jacket, hood and sunglasses. Tears for my donor and his family, tears of the fear of failure and tears of determination.' But, with help from the group's doctor, he pressed on and two days later reached 5,895 m – the summit. 'His heart and I had made it' ...

At forty-seven, Ernesto still has other heights to conquer. Why does he push himself so hard? 'I do it for my donor,' he says simply, 'and to inspire others to join the Organ Donor Register.'

Both Kate and Ernesto have been present during retrieval surgery when organs are removed from cadaver donors. They fear that the general public's perception of how organs are retrieved is very much misguided. 'The utmost dignity is given to both donors and their families at all times as they have given the ultimate gift – the gift of life.'

Jade's Story

'A Normal, Lively Little Girl'

When 7-year-old Jade Stoner was lying fatally injured in a hospital bed relatives flew in from Canada and Dubai to sit with her and say goodbye. 'As soon as they heard they took the first flights they could get to be there in time,' says Jade's mother, Debbie, 'and the doctors were happy for her to remain on life support until they could get there. There was no rush or pressure from the hospital and my brother sat beside the bed for an hour.'

It was a Sunday afternoon, in September 2006, when Jade was knocked off her bicycle right outside the family home on the outskirts of Christchurch, Dorset. She was taken first to Bournemouth Hospital, where Debbie and her husband, John, were told there was little hope. Soon after she was transferred to Poole Hospital for continued life support. The question of donation came up and, says Debbie, 'The staff there were brilliant. They didn't put any pressure on us and gave us all the time we needed.

'In the end, all Jade's organs were donated except the lungs and eyes. We had a card from one of the recipients just before Christmas to say he was doing well.'

Meanwhile, 4-year-old Amy had witnessed her sister's accident. 'Amy said she knew Jade was dead straight away. She began having nightmares and had trouble sleeping. She told me she didn't want to talk about the accident at first in case she upset the rest of us,' said Debbie.

Jade's 15-year-old half-brother, James, was also deeply affected and Debbie sought some counselling for the family. 'But my mum, who's a counsellor herself, was so concerned about the lack of help for bereaved people that she wrote a letter about the accident in the local paper and that brought in a huge response – lots of letters and e-mails. So then we decided to start our own bereavement counselling group in Bournemouth. We didn't know what to expect at the first meeting but loads of people turned up. The place was packed.

'Jade was just a normal, lively little girl who loved things that were pink and glittery. Losing her left a great big hole in all our lives.'

John's Story

'It was Hard to Take in at First'

Linda Edwards cannot speak too highly of the nursing and medical staff she met when her husband was dying. 'They were kindness itself,' she says, 'and we never felt we were being pressured. Not before he died, not afterwards when we knew they had to act within minutes or the organs would go to waste.'

John and Linda had been married for twenty-three years and had one son, Matthew, then aged 12. Linda's surprise present for John's fiftieth birthday had been a four-day trip to celebrate in New York just two weeks previously. Then, one Saturday evening in June 2007, Matthew went into the hall and found his father collapsed on the floor. He was taken first to the Mayday Hospital in Croydon, where they hinted his chances were poor, and then, within a few hours, on to the Atkinson Morley Wing at St George's Hospital in south London.

The following morning the consultant confirmed that John had suffered a subarachnoid haemorrhage and that there was no hope; the damage had been too great. Linda said: 'It was hard to take it on at first, what with the shock and the speed at which things were happening, but I knew what to do when they raised the question of donation. I'd carried a donor card for years but John hadn't and we'd never discussed it. Matthew and I talked it over and we felt we probably should donate his organs.

'The doctors and nurses insisted that I could change my mind if I wanted to right up to the last minute but I wanted to know at what point the intended recipients would be told that organs had been found for them. I didn't want them getting their hopes up and then having them dashed, and me having the burden of guilt on top of everything else. I was 99 per cent sure I was doing the right thing, that John would have gone along with it. He was a logical man and a kind man ...'

John was not brainstem-dead but instead became what is known as a non-heartbeating donor (see Chapter 3). Towards the end most of the monitoring equipment was removed and John was taken to a side room in the theatre suite where he died on the Monday evening. Linda will always be grateful to the woman doctor who, when she was about to send Matthew home, suggested it might help him to stay. 'I'm so glad he was there because it was so peaceful, and when his dad passed away he leaned over and kissed him on the forehead.

'It sounds funny to say but there was a very peaceful atmosphere in that room. At the end, when I looked behind me, I saw that my family had been joined by the transplant co-ordinator and the intensive care nurse who had been looking after John. But even then there was no pressure because we'd been prepared, we'd had time to say our private goodbyes and now we knew they'd want to move quickly once John's heart had stopped.'

The transplant co-ordinator later wrote to Linda to say that four recipients had been grafted from her husband's donation of liver, both kidneys and one of the heart valves. 'What I really appreciated was that she went to the trouble of writing two letters: one to me and a separate one to Matthew in language that a 12-year-old would be able to understand.'

Laura's Story

Chasing the Mirage

Laura Fasching's story is a harrowing one since, for her as for many other chronically sick youngsters, good health was to remain a mirage. Laura was born with liver disease, had her first liver transplant at the age of eleven months, suffered innumerable grave illnesses and by her tenth year was diagnosed with a further serious liver disease. She continued on this roller-coaster for more than a decade and for the most part was unwilling to discuss her illness. 'I hate it when people ask me how I am,' she would say. 'What do I tell them? "Fine?" All I want is to get well, be with my friends and get my life back.'

For Laura's parents – Helena, who comes from Colombia, and Austrian-born Peter – it was an uphill struggle from day one. They recall having to trek her, as a jaundiced newborn, round four different London hospitals for an accurate diagnosis. Helena said: 'Right from the start I knew there was something wrong but all that happened was that I gained a reputation as an anxious mother. I can remember in one hospital in the East End sitting for days on end alone with Laura in a cubicle. In the end they sent us on to the Queen Elizabeth Hospital in Hackney, where they found it was a problem with the liver. Fortunately the registrar there had worked on the liver unit at King's College Hospital and so he transferred us there.'

In south London, King's confirmed the diagnosis: Laura, by now turned two months of age and still jaundiced, had biliary atresia, a congenital condition in which the ducts draining bile from the liver are blocked or missing. The trouble is that corrective surgery for biliary atresia (the Kasai procedure) needs to be done within eight weeks of birth to have the best chance of success. Because of the delay in diagnosing Laura's condition, she could not undergo surgery until she was nine weeks old. The operation was unsuccessful and bile continued to accumulate, causing further damage to the liver.

Helena said: 'Laura was sick most of the time, with permanent cholangitis (inflammation of the bile ducts), which meant that she was hardly ever at home.' By the age of six months she was on nasogastric feeding and after another two months, her abdomen distended with fluid (ascites), she was being assessed for transplantation. The operation took place at Addenbrooke's Hospital in Cambridge in December 1989. 'Within a week,' says her mother, 'she was sitting up in bed eating everything she could get hold of.'

However, the post-operative course was stormy and Laura had to remain in hospital for five long months. There was another setback ten months after the transplant, necessitating further surgery. After this Laura made good progress and remained well until she was 7 years old, when she suddenly came down with a serious infection. This led to acute kidney failure and a further stay in intensive care. Again she made a full recovery.

The next blow came when, at the age of 10, Laura was diagnosed with liver disease: autoimmune hepatitis. She still recalls the 'roid rages' (aggressive outbursts) brought on by the steroids used to treat it. She battled this condition – the most severe of the chronic forms of hepatitis – throughout her secondary school career, having good days and bad. Even so, the following year she was able to enjoy a week-long trip to the Seychelles, laid on for her by the Make-A-Wish Foundation UK, an organisation which works to make good things happen for children with life-threatening diseases.

The next five years or so were relatively tranquil, but then, when Laura was in her mid teens, her condition began to deteriorate once again. In the space of a few days she blew up like a balloon owing to the accumulation of fluid that is a feature of advanced liver disease. Laura, of course, has no recollection of the events which followed. Over the course of the next two months the family watched as she drifted in and out of consciousness, put on a staggering 25 kg (55 lb) in weight, suffered several bouts of hospital-acquired infection (including the dreaded MRSA) and one or two episodes of kidney shutdown. She also had to undergo surgery to deal with a potentially lethal narrowing of the abdominal aorta, the body's main artery. Then, inexplicably, came the day when she suddenly lost 4 litres (7 pints) of fluid in two hours ...

Miraculously, Laura survived this horrific illness and, as she began to recover, was put on the waiting list for a new liver. She later took herself off the list, in what she conceded was a bid to take back control of her life, but reluctantly agreed to go back on it after a few months. For a while Laura worked at various jobs – as an au pair, waitress and intern in an architects' practice. But, coming from an artistic family, she hoped to make a career in fashion journalism and so, in September 2009, she began a course at the University College for the Creative Arts in Epsom, Surrey.

Never really well, Laura managed to keep up with the course until one night in December, when she was found at 2.00 a.m. lying unconscious in a corridor at the halls of residence. She was taken first to Epsom General Hospital and then on to King's College Hospital, where she spent a week in intensive care with a suspected liver infection. Back in Epsom after the Christmas holidays, she struggled on for another few weeks with the help of a carer and an alarm button in her room for use in an emergency. In March she made her way home to Cambridge for Mother's Day. 'As the day went on she seemed uncertain about going back,' says Helena, 'and in the end she decided to stay here because she was very tired and sleeping most of the time.' At home she became steadily worse and finally, on 17 March 2010, she had to be taken back into Addenbrooke's in excruciating pain.

Admitted with a liver infection, she then went on to develop pneumonia and spent two days in intensive care. Weathering yet another crisis she was transferred back to the liver unit, but subsequently had several visits to the hospital's high-dependency unit with recurrent bouts of mental confusion (hepatic encephalopathy) caused by the sick liver's failure to clear the body of toxic substances. The waiting, of course, seemed interminable and the chronic anxiety was affecting Laura's whole family: her parents and her sister, Hannah, aged 19, and 12-year-old brother, Maxi. The average waiting time for a new liver in this country is about five months and so Laura's predicament was exceptional, not least because at barely 4 foot 11 inches she was too small for most of the adult livers becoming available. At present in Britain 10–15 per cent of people on the liver transplant waiting list are dying before a new liver becomes available and the (largely unspoken) fear in the Fasching household was that Laura, too, would die or become too ill for a transplant.

For almost six months Laura's life was on hold for, although she could be driven the few miles home for a couple of hours most days, it would have been unsafe for her to leave hospital. The frequent crises which occur in end-stage liver disease are potentially fatal ones, needing rapid access to resuscitation facilities and intensive care. Laura knew all this, having lived with liver disease since birth. In twenty-one years she had experienced virtually all the complications known to hepatology, including: nausea and vomiting; itching; jaundice; gall stones; vomiting blood; massive fluid retention; acute kidney failure; and encephalopathy. So by early September, brought low by repeated crises during a prolonged hospital stay, she no longer cared whether she lived or died. 'On the day before the transplant I was about to take myself off the waiting list,' she admitted. 'I just wanted it all to end. But then we got this phone call ...'

When it came to it, Laura's second liver transplant, on 9 September 2010, turned into a nineteen-hour surgical marathon – an operation made more difficult because of all the previous interventions. Perhaps not surprisingly, the post-operative course was also difficult, with two further visits to theatre for the surgeons to deal with bleeding and treatment for acute kidney shutdown. Laura meanwhile wrote to her donor's family within a few days of surgery. 'I felt I had to do it as soon as I was able.' During the interim period, she and the family were heartened by two visits to the bedside by the eminent surgeon, now retired, who had carried out the first transplant.

Laura now enjoyed what recipients sometimes refer to as the honeymoon period of unaccustomed good health following a transplant. But again the mirage receded. She started to go downhill once more and at length, on Christmas Day 2010, she had to be carried into hospital – sick and hopelessly weak, her body already ballooning with fluid. Acute rejection had set in, soon followed by pneumonia, failing kidneys and a host of other complications, each one a fresh challenge for the intensive care staff battling to save her life. Finally, surrounded by presents and cards from well-wishers on her twenty-second birthday, Laura went into cardiac arrest and died.

Martin's Story

'Thank God I was There'

There are two things in particular that continue to bring some comfort to Sue Burton more than eight years after the sudden loss of her younger son. One is that she was in the house when Martin collapsed and the other is the knowledge that his organs saved or enhanced the lives of eight people. Aged 16, Martin was a real boy – 'noisy, boisterous and into everything', according to his mother. He had recently left school and, wanting to train as a nurse, he was due to enrol at the local college the following day.

The night it happened, late in August 2003, Martin and his mother were alone in the house. His father, Nigel, at that time in the RAF, was away in the US; the couple's older son, Chris, then aged 20, was staying at his girlfriend's house. It was 2.00 a.m. when Sue heard some crashes and thuds and then Martin appeared in her bedroom doorway. 'I asked him if he was alright and he looked at me with a glazed, confused expression. I realised later his brain was shutting down. He probably couldn't see or hear me and he certainly couldn't speak. He staggered towards my bed and collapsed onto it. Then he rolled over and fell on the floor.'

Martin was taken first to the local hospital then on to the Queen's Medical Centre in Nottingham, arriving at 5.00 a.m. Sue was told three hours later there was nothing more to be done – Martin was brainstem-dead. It seemed he had been born with a rare congenital abnormality of some blood vessels in the brain (arteriovenous malformation) and that this had burst, resulting in a massive haemorrhage.

The consultant asked if Sue would consider donating Martin's organs. 'I said yes immediately. Although we had never discussed it, I was sure Nigel would go along with it and I believe Martin would have wanted it, too. I thought if I could save one other mother from going through the nightmare of losing someone, it would be worth it.

'You have to sign an agreement for each individual organ. You can say yes to some and no to others, and you also decide, if the organs aren't fit to be used, whether you want them left in the body or taken for research. I've never seen the donation as a violation of Martin's body but I suppose I felt at the time that letting his organs go for research would be.'

Martin was maintained on life support until his father could make the long journey home. Sue sat at the bedside until Nigel arrived the following morning and later that day the couple said their goodbyes. 'I didn't want to see Martin go so the transplant co-ordinator accompanied him to theatre for me. The hardest moment for me was walking out of that hospital leaving my son behind.

'The whole thing was a nightmare but, thank God, if it had to happen it was at night and I was there, not out at work or something. I hope he knew that I was there with him, that he wasn't alone.' Sue and Nigel have since become trustees of Donor Family Network (see Useful Organisations at the back of this book), anxious to use their experience to help others.

Martin became a multi-organ donor. Sue said, 'We're thrilled to have updates from the transplant co-ordinator and to hear how well the recipients are doing, particularly the 15-year-old boy who received Martin's heart. It's strange to think that his heart is still beating somewhere ... Now we more often think of Martin with a smile rather than tears. Our love for him is as strong as ever but we are learning to integrate our loss as part of our lives rather than it being the all-consuming whole of our lives.'

Rick's Story

'There's Nothing We Can Do'

Liz Phillips wasn't particularly flustered when they rang from the football club to say her husband had collapsed on the field. At age 38 – 'They called him the old man' – Richard (Rick) Phillips was still playing for his works team regularly each week but one of his knees had been playing up. Busy cooking lunch for the extended family, Liz recalls, 'I thought they were going to say he'd broken his leg.'

While Rick had been alert and talking on the football field, he was unconscious by the time Liz saw him in Warrington Hospital. 'He'd had a scan and they told me he'd had a slight bleed in the brain and they'd had to put him on a machine to help his breathing. They were going to send him to the Fazakerley Hospital in Liverpool because the specialists there thought they might be able to help him.'

A father of four, Rick had always been very fit except for a brief spell a fortnight previously. 'He suddenly came over poorly. I remember he had trouble getting off the sofa to get over to the window. He said he'd feel better if he could get a breath of fresh air. I've often wondered whether that was the start of it.'

When Liz got to the Fazakerley Rick had been taken to theatre, where they discovered that the 'slight bleed' had in fact been a massive one. 'There was this chap in blue theatre kit who said to me, "I don't know why they sent him to us. There's nothing we can do." They'd tried obviously, because when he came out of theatre there was a bandage round his head with blood on it. I could feel his feet were cold and the coldness seemed to go further up his legs as time went on.

'They came and talked to us about organ donation and did the brainstem death tests on the Wednesday.' By a strange coincidence, a couple of weeks before Rick's death he and Liz had seen a TV programme about organ donation. 'He said, "If anything happens to me they can have my organs." And I said, "You can't do that. Supposing I went to the graveside to talk to you. There wouldn't be all of you there." And he said, "Well, I won't be in the cemetery because I want to be cremated." So we agreed that it was better for his organs to go to help others rather than be burned up.

'That was a hard thing to tell the children but my sister and her husband and I sat down with them in the garden and talked the whole thing through so they could be part of it. They all said what they wanted for the funeral and they chose the music. The only thing I did ask the undertakers was not to have the coffin start moving while we were still in the chapel. I wanted them just to leave the curtains open and wait till we'd gone outside.'

Liz and the children moved down to Nottinghamshire less than a year later in order to be close to Rick's family. Sadly, since her father's death Jade, the youngest of the four children, has developed health problems, including autoimmune liver disease. Several years ago she underwent major surgery, but with support from an unexpected quarter – the man who received her dad's liver. Liz said: 'I'm so glad he has befriended her because it helps to hear from someone else who has had the same kind of problems, especially since the hospital have told us that sooner or later it could mean a liver transplant. She's fine at the moment, hoping to train as a paediatric nurse.

'If ever I was in two minds about organ donation I'm all for it now with my own daughter likely to need a new liver. So, you see, we'll have experienced it from both sides.'

Tineke's Story

A Glowing Advert

Aged 38, Tineke Dixon is a glowing advert for transplantation for she started life as a 'blue baby' who was not expected to live to adulthood. Today, as one of the longest-surviving heart-lung recipients – she was transplanted at the age of 16 – she holds down a key position in NHS financial management and runs her own 30 ft racing yacht. She owes her survival and obvious good health to four donated organs: a heart-lung block from a deceased donor and a kidney from her mother.

Tineke says she was born 'a congenital disaster zone', with a heart malformation which gives rise to the rare and debilitating condition known as Eisenmenger's syndrome. Tied for much of her childhood to a wheelchair and oxygen cylinder, she suffered unremitting fatigue, breathlessness and a general failure to thrive. At the age of 16, lying in Great Ormond Street Hospital, she was given six months to live. 'I can still remember hearing my parents' cries of anguish coming down a corridor as the doctors told them how little time I had left.'

She was told that her only hope lay in a heart-lung transplant, then still very much an experimental procedure. 'It was touch and go really. Two other youngsters who had similar operations before me at Great Ormond Street sadly died after a few years. I really count myself very lucky indeed.'

The six-hour operation took place at Great Ormond Street Hospital in London in November 1988 and Tineke soon gained sufficient ground to embark on a degree course in medical physics at Exeter University. She went on to do a PhD in Cambridge and then started working in IT in the radiology department at Addenbrooke's Hospital in Cambridge.

But by 1996 Tineke found she had inherited the polycystic kidney disease which had plagued her father for years – he'd had a kidney transplant five years earlier – and by now her kidneys were failing. After a frustrating two years on dialysis she was transplanted with a kidney donated by her mother in December 1998. The operation, she says, was 'easy compared with a heart-lung transplant', and she has remained well ever since. She moved back to the West Country seven years later, not least to spend more time sailing.

The year 2008 was a momentous one for Tineke because, besides getting married to Clive, she was also able to celebrate two anniversaries: twenty years for the heart-lung graft and ten years for the kidney. 'There's no doubt I'd have been pushing up the daisies by the time I was 16 or 17 if it hadn't been for the new heart and lungs. They told me in 1988 that it wouldn't last long, that I was breaking new ground. There aren't many of us around with donated organs over 20 years old.'

Tineke has had episodes of rejection and infection in the past but is more stable now. Both transplants were good matches, she believes. 'I haven't taken any steroids for years and I'm on a comparatively low dose of immunosuppression. I suppose there could be stuff going on inside me but I don't dwell on what *might* happen. I feel perfectly fine and I'm determined to live life to the full.' Based in Exmouth, she and Clive spend as much time as possible out on the water. The summer of 2010 was a bumper one, with a win in their class in the club sailing, taking three trophies, and a creditable sixth place in the Dartmouth Regatta on their first time there.

'I often think about the woman who donated her heart and lungs to me, and her family, of course, and I am very grateful to them. If I live an honourable and useful life I feel I am paying them back for their gift.'

Glossary

Acute	The term used to describe a medical condition of sudden and severe onset but which resolves quickly. In contrast, a chronic condition develops and remains over a long period.
Allograft	The transfer of living tissue from one individual to another of the same species, as in blood transfusion or organ transplantation.
Anastomosis	A connection between two vessels in the body. Surgical anastomosis involves the joining of two sections of a vessel (such as reuniting each end of a severed blood vessel) or hollow parts of an organ as, for example, when a section of intestine has been removed and the remaining free ends are brought together and stitched.
Antibody	Protein produced in the blood by lymphocytes in response to the presence of foreign or invading substances (antigens, see below). By binding to the antigen, antibody enhances the immune response to foreign cells.
Antigen	Any substance, like a toxin or other foreign substance, which causes the production of antibodies by the body's immune system. The proteins of incompatible blood groups or tissues also act as antigens.

Apnoea	The absence of or temporary cessation of spontaneous breathing movements. In brainstem death apnoea is irreversible. It means that the respiratory centre in the brain has ceased to function and the person is incapable of breathing independently when the ventilator is disconnected.
Asystole	Condition in which the chambers of the heart fail to contract. The patient loses consciousness immediately but may continue to breathe spontaneously for up to sixty seconds. No pulse can be felt at the arteries and no heart sounds are heard. The electrocardiogram registers a 'flat' line (see also cardiac arrest, below). The non-heartbeating donor is sometimes referred to as an asystolic donor.
Atresia	The congenital absence or abnormal narrowing of a body opening or duct. Biliary atresia, in which the ducts draining bile from the liver are blocked or missing, is the commonest condition requiring liver transplantation in children.
Autograft	Tissue taken from one part of the body for grafting at another part of the same person, as in the repair of burns.
Biopsy	Removal of a sample of tissue from a living body for examination to determine presence, cause or extent of a disease. It is common for transplanted organs to be biopsied to investigate rejection.
Brainstem	Stalk at the base of the brain where it merges with the spinal cord. It is the site of the vital centres maintaining the body's own life-support system: breathing, heartbeat, blood pressure and level of consciousness. All information between the body and the brain is relayed through the brainstem.

Cardiac arrest	Sudden failure of the heart's pumping action. It may cease to beat altogether (asystole, see above) or go into a rapid, chaotic rhythm. The person loses consciousness and stops breathing. Without resuscitation death follows within minutes.
Cardiomyopathy	Chronic disorder or disease of the heart muscle. It may be inherited or it may arise from a range of conditions, including infection. The condition may cause enlargement of the heart as well as heart failure and disruption of the heart rhythm.
Catheter	A flexible tube inserted into the body to introduce or remove fluids. A urinary catheter is passed through the urethra into the bladder to drain urine into a collecting bag.
Cerebral cortex	The outer layer of the brain, the 'grey matter' which is responsible for all conscious function and voluntary activity.
Cirrhosis	A degenerative condition in an organ of the body, especially the liver, characterised by scarring and painful swelling. It may arise from a number of causes. When the liver is affected it becomes enlarged, hard and knobbly. Untreated, it can progress to coma and death.
Collagen	A protein that is the main constituent of animal connective tissue (see below). Collagen is present in skin, cartilage, tendons and ligaments. Bones are made up of collagen, with the mineral calcium phosphate providing increased rigidity.
Coma	A state of unconsciousness from which the person cannot be roused.

Congenital — Used to describe any condition which is present at birth. It may be inherited from the parents or it may occur as a result of some environmental factor.

Connective tissue — Tissue that connects, supports, binds or separates other tissues or organs. Consists of a non-cellular substance, the extracellular matrix, in which some cells are embedded. Skin, bones, tendons, cartilage and adipose tissue (fat) are the main connective tissues. There are also small amounts of connective tissue in organs such as the brain and liver, where they give the organ shape and structure.

Cortiscosteroid — Any of a group of steroid hormones produced in the adrenal cortex, which is the outer substance of the endocrine gland located on the top surface of each kidney. Corticosteroids play key roles in a number of physiological functions, including metabolism and the immune response. Synthetic corticosteroids are used in medical treatment, including immuno-suppressive therapy.

Cystic fibrosis — An inherited disease which affects the lungs, pancreas and digestive tract. It leads to repeated severe lung infections and progressive damage to the airways. Some patients who are severely affected benefit from double-lung transplants. Because of increased life expectancy, some adults with this condition develop liver disease as a late complication.

DBD — Abbreviation for donation after brainstem death.

DCD — Abbreviation for organ donation following cardiac death – that is, after the heart has stopped.

Dialysis — A technique for removing toxic waste products from the blood of someone in kidney failure. Blood is passed across a fine membrane and waste products

	filter through into a dialysing solution on the other side of the membrane. There are two methods: haemodialysis, by way of the artificial kidney machine, and peritoneal dialysis, which makes use of the tissue lining the abdomen as the dialysing membrane.
Diuretic	Any drug that increases the output of urine from the kidneys.
Domino procedure	The use of a healthy heart, removed from a patient receiving a heart-lung transplant, to save a patient in heart failure. In practice, since so few heart-lung transplants are performed these days, domino grafts are exceedingly rare. Occasionally, too, a domino liver can be performed following transplantation of the liver for metabolic disease (see Chapter 5).
DTC	Abbreviation for donor transplant co-ordinator (see SNOD).
Embryo	The term embryo describes the fertilised egg during the first seven weeks of its existence; from the eighth week it is known as a fetus.
End-stage organ disease	Condition where failure of an organ becomes irreversible.
ESRD	Abbreviation for end-stage renal disease.
Graft	An organ or tissue transplanted to replace a part of the body which is damaged or non-functioning.
Hepatectomy	Surgical removal of the liver.
Hepatic	Of or pertaining to the liver.
Hepatocyte	The principal functional cell of the liver.

Heterotopic	An adjective used to describe a graft implanted elsewhere than in its normal anatomical position; for instance, the transplanted kidney positioned within the pelvis.
HLA	Abbreviation for the human leucocyte antigen system, a series of gene groups that code for proteins on the surface of cells. If two people have the same HLA types they are said to be histocompatible: that is, they are a good match for transplantation.
Hypoglycaemia	A condition of an abnormally low level of sugar (glucose) in the blood, which starves the brain. It causes weakness, sweating, confusion, sometimes fainting. Uncorrected, it would lead to coma and death. Hypoglycaemia is most often seen in people with diabetes.
Immune system	Complex set of mechanisms which protects the body against infection, maintains a constant internal environment and guards against abnormalities.
Immunodeficient	Lacking one or more elements of a working immune system. Immune deficiency is the term generally used for people who are born with such a defect, while those who acquire the condition later in life (such as transplant recipients) are referred to as being immunocompromised or immunosuppressed.
Immuno-suppressant	A drug which suppresses the body's immune responses.
Infusion	A slow injection of a drug or other therapeutic substance into the body.

Intensive care unit (ICU)	Specialised hospital facility which treats people with life-threatening conditions. Patients who have had major surgery, such as a heart, lung or liver transplant, are taken to intensive care post-operatively for observation, monitoring and support. Less often the term intensive therapy unit (ITU) is used.
Ischaemia	Reduction of blood supply (and therefore vital oxygen) to any part of the body. It results in damage to and ultimately death of tissues and organs.
Islet cell	A cell from one of the groups of cells within the pancreas, known as the islets of Langerhans, which secrete the hormone insulin.
Jaundice	A yellow discoloration of the skin and whites of the eyes which is caused by an excess of bile pigment in the bloodstream. The causes include some types of anaemia, liver disease or gallstones. The jaundice recedes following treatment.
Kaposi's sarcoma	A malignant tumour developing from blood vessels in the skin. Previously rare in the developed world, it is now seen in some patients with AIDS and in some transplant recipients.
Laparoscope	An instrument used for 'keyhole' investigation or surgery. It consists of an illuminated viewing tube with its own attachments and an inbuilt camera linked to a viewing screen.
Larynx	The cavity at the upper end of the windpipe (trachea) which contains the vocal cords. It is stiffened with cartilage and lined with mucous membrane.
Leucocyte	Another name for a white blood cell involved in counteracting foreign substances and infection.

Lymphocyte A type of white blood cell with a single large nucleus which is produced in the bone marrow. Lymphocytes are present in the blood and lymph and also in the spleen, thymus gland and intestinal wall. B-lymphocytes are responsible for producing antibodies (see above); T-cells have various roles in the mechanism of immunity.

Lymphoma Any malignant tumour of the lymph nodes.

Melanoma A highly malignant tumour of the melanin-forming cells (melanocytes) of the skin. In most cases it develops from an existing mole, but it can also arise in the eyes or mucous membranes. Associated with excessive exposure to sunlight, it is the most dangerous of the skin cancers – easily treated if caught early but deadly once it has spread. Transplant recipients are at particular risk of melanoma.

Metabolism Term used for the sum of all the chemical and physical changes taking place within the body to enable its continued growth, maintenance and repair. By digestion the body partially breaks down complex organic substances, ingested as food, and subsequently re-synthesises them for its own purposes.

Monoclonal antibody (MAB) An antibody produced artificially by fusing an antibody-producing lymphocyte from mouse spleen with a cancerous myeloma (bone marrow), also from a mouse. The resulting fused cell, called a hybridoma, is immortal and can be used to produce large quantities of a single, specific antibody. MABs are used for research and diagnostic investigation and have also been developed as therapeutic agents to treat a variety of conditions, including rejection.

Multi-organ donor A person who, at death, donates several organs for transplantation.

Nasogastric tube	A flexible tube which is passed through the nose and down the oesophagus into the stomach. It is used to introduce fluids (in particular liquid food) into the stomach or sometimes to empty it.
Nephrectomy	The surgical removal of one or both kidneys, often done by keyhole surgery (see laparoscope above).
Nephrotoxic	Harmful to the kidneys. Some drugs, including some used in transplantation, are nephrotoxic.
Neuron(e)	Another name for a nerve cell.
NICE	Abbreviation for the National Institute for Health and Clinical Excellence – the body set up in 1999 to promote high-quality and cost-effective treatments and services within the NHS. It defines standards of care, issues guidance on best practice and on disease prevention and the promotion of health. NICE also aims to reduce regional discrepancies in NHS care.
Oedema	Any abnormal accumulation of fluid in the tissues or cavities of the body. It may be generalised (the condition once known as dropsy) or confined to one area, such as the ankles.
Osteoporosis	The condition in which there is loss of bony tissue, making bones brittle and liable to break. The generalised condition is seen mostly in post-menopausal women and the elderly, but osteoporosis can occur in other circumstances, including as a result of prolonged steroid therapy.
Pancreas	A large accessory gland of the digestive system located close to the duodenum and behind and below the stomach. When stimulated by the hormone secretin, the pancreas releases enzymes into the duodenum that digest starches, proteins and fats. About 18 cm (7 in) in

length in the adult, it contains groups of cells called the islets of Langerhans, which secrete the hormones insulin and glucagon that regulate the blood-sugar level.

Paediatrics — The medical specialty concerned with the diseases of childhood.

Parenteral — Adjective describing the introduction of drugs and other substances by any route other than by mouth. Parenteral fluids are delivered using a drip.

Pathogen — Commonly called a germ, the term pathogen is applied to any micro-organism, such as a bacterium or virus, that causes disease. Transplant recipients and others with depressed immune systems are at risk from some pathogens which are harmless to most people, such as bacteria which live in the soil or in the gut.

Plasma — The liquid component of the blood in which the blood cells are suspended.

PKD — Abbreviation for polycystic kidney disease, a hereditary condition associated with chronic kidney failure.

Rejection — Immune response to donor tissue. If it goes unchecked, the graft is destroyed. Acute rejection develops rapidly, usually from one week to several months after transplantation, but mostly it can be reversed with drug treatment. Chronic rejection, a slow, insidious process resulting in gradual impairment of the transplanted organ, is irreversible.

Renal — Of or pertaining to the kidney.

Roid rage — A term used for hostile or downright aggressive outbursts sometimes seen in people taking high doses of steroids.

RRT — Abbreviation for renal replacement therapy.

Segmental graft	Transplant using only a segment, or part, of an organ. Liver segmental grafts (fashioned from adult organs) increase the number of donor livers available to transplant into babies and small children.
Sepsis	A general term for infectious changes in tissues in the body caused by harmful bacteria or their toxins, typically through the infection of a wound.
SNOD	Abbreviation for a specialist nurse in organ donation, formerly known as a donor transplant co-ordinator.
SPK	Abbreviation for a simultaneous pancreas-kidney transplant.
Tissue bank	Centre for storage of donated tissues, such as corneas, blood, bone and bone marrow.
Tissue typing	Laboratory tests to determine leucocyte (white blood cell) type. Donor and recipient tissues are matched to improve the chances of a successful transplant.
Total parenteral nutrition (TPN)	The use of intravenous feeding for patients who are unable to absorb nutrients from a normal diet.
Trachea	The medical term for the windpipe. It runs from the larynx to the upper part of the chest, then branches into two tubes, the left and right bronchi, conveying air to the lungs.
Vegetative state	Condition arising from overwhelming damage to the cerebral cortex. The patient lies unresponsive and, though the eyes may be open, he or she has no awareness of the surroundings, makes no purposeful gestures, shows no voluntary response to stimuli and never speaks. The vegetative patient may survive for many years in a condition which many observers regard as a living death.

Ventilator	A machine to assist breathing or to take over when the patient is unable to breathe unaided. The lungs are inflated with a mixture of oxygen and air. As long as the person's heart continues to beat, oxygen is picked up by the blood and carried to all the tissues throughout the body.
Xenotransplantation	The grafting of a tissue or organ from one species into another. Most xenografts performed on human beings provoke very severe rejection.

Historical Milestones

1901 In Vienna, Karl Landsteiner reported the discovery of ABO blood groups. Compatibility of blood groups is important for successful transfusion and tissue and organ grafting.

1902 Alexis Carrel demonstrated a method of joining blood vessels together (anastomosis), a surgical technique which is essential for transplantation.

1905 Austrian surgeon Eduard Zirm performed the first corneal transplant in Olmutz, Moravia (now the Czech Republic).

1918 In World War I, blood transfusion became established practice.

1923 In the US, Carl Williamson examined a failed kidney graft, described its appearance and coined the term 'rejection'.

1937 Russian surgeon Yu Yu Voronoy attempted transplantation of an unmatched cadaver kidney; the organ failed to work.

1943 Peter Medawar and colleagues showed that the rejection of skin allografts (from one person to another) is an immunological phenomenon.

1948 Foundation of the National Health Service.

1954 The first successful kidney transplant carried out in Boston, Massachusetts. Ronald Herrick donated a kidney to his identical twin, Richard, who lived for a further eight years.

1955 First successful heart-lung machine developed in Minnesota. This became a powerful tool for transplant surgeons, enabling major procedures where the circulation is interrupted.

1958 Total body irradiation first used in Paris to suppress the immune reaction to transplanted organs.

1959 Two French neurologists defined the condition *coma dépassé* – a state beyond coma, which in the UK came to be known as brainstem death.

1960 The UK's first living donor kidney transplant performed in Edinburgh.

1962 First reports of the anti-rejection drug azathioprine in the US.

1963 First liver transplant carried out in Denver, Colorado.

1963 First successful lung transplant reported at the University of Mississippi.

1963 Reports of thirteen kidney transplants using organs from chimpanzees; the longest recorded survival is nine months.

1965 The UK's first kidney transplant from a non-heartbeating donor took place in Edinburgh.

1966 Report of the first prospective trial of human leucocyte antigen (HLA) matching for donor selection in the US.

1966 First pancreas transplant reported from Minnesota.

1967 In South Africa Christiaan Barnard performed the first heart transplant.

1968 First UK heart transplant; the recipient died from infection nine weeks later.

1968 First UK liver transplant.

1968 The world's first multi-organ donor was a Texas woman who died from a gunshot wound to the head.

1971 The kidney donor card was introduced in the UK; ten years later it became the organ donor card.

1971 The need for better understanding of rejection became a factor in the establishment of the British Transplantation Society.

1976 Brainstem death protocols introduced in UK.

1977 Ciclosporin shown to be a powerful immunosuppressant. First used in the UK the following year.

1979 The National Tissue Typing and Reference Laboratory (set up in 1968) and the 7-year-old National Organ Matching and Distribution Service merged to form the UK Transplant Service.

1983 First UK combined heart-lung transplant, two years after the procedure was pioneered at Stanford University in the US.

1983 The first successful single lung transplant carried out at the University of Toronto.

1984 Baby Fae received a baboon heart at Loma Linda University in California. She survived for twenty days, succumbing to kidney failure. There was no sign that her body had rejected the heart.

1988 The first prolonged survival following combined liver-small bowel transplant reported from the University of Western Ontario.

1991 UK Transplant Service renamed the United Kingdom Transplant Support Service Authority (UKTSSA).

1994 First dual organ transplant (pancreas and kidney) from a living donor carried out in Minnesota.

1994 The new immunosuppressive drug FK506 (tacrolimus) licensed for use in the US. It has a similar mode of action to that of ciclosporin but is more powerful and in some ways more toxic.

1994 The NHS Organ Donor Register (ODR) established.

1994 First UK living donor liver transplant.

1995 First UK living donor lung (lobe) transplant.

1998 First successful hand transplant carried out in Lyon, France.

1999 Researchers at the University of Alberta in Edmonton, Canada, developed techniques to collect and prepare pancreatic islet cells for transplantation. The 'Edmonton protocol' was taken up by centres around the world.

2000 UKTSSA became UK Transplant.

2001 First non-heartbeating lung transplant carried out in Lund, Sweden.

2005 UK Transplant merged with National Blood Service to form NHS Blood and Transplant (NHSBT).

2005 First partial face transplant carried out at Amiens in France.

2006 Surgeons reversed the heart transplant of a 12-year-old girl from south Wales. In heart failure a decade earlier, she had been given a 'piggyback' heart which had enabled her own heart to recover.

2008 Surgeons in New Jersey pioneered the first robot-assisted kidney transplant.

2010 Ronald Herrick, who had donated a kidney to his twin brother Richard 56 years previously, died at the age of 79.

Appendix I

Testing for Brainstem Death

The UK protocols for diagnosing death of the brainstem incorporate simple tests which can be carried out at the bedside. These tests explore the viability of the brainstem – the body's own life-support centre – in two ways. In the first place they establish whether or not certain nerve reflexes are working for, as an eminent British neurologist has pointed out, testing these reflexes 'probes the brainstem slice by slice, as if it were salami'. In addition, there is a test to determine whether or not the comatose patient can breathe unaided.

By no means all ventilated patients in deep coma are candidates for testing. Some do not meet the preconditions laid down in the UK code of practice because their unconscious state has developed from a cause which is potentially reversible. In this category are those whose coma is as a result of the prolonged effects of some drugs, to hypothermia or to some gross disturbance of body chemistry. Cases which meet the preconditions are those arising from a known cause of irreversible damage, including: head injury, brain haemorrhage, primary brain tumour or failure of the oxygen supply to the brain as, for example, in suffocation.

Once an unconscious patient is admitted to intensive care, the length of time he or she remains on life-support depends on the cause of the coma. Normally, brainstem death would not be considered as a possible diagnosis until at least six hours have elapsed; often the interval is much longer.

When the coma persists, the code calls for testing to be undertaken by two experienced medical staff – either two consultants or a consultant and a senior trainee – neither of whom have anything to do with transplantation. First, they try to elicit the reflexes which signal life in the brainstem. This is done by:

1) Shining a light into each of the patient's eyes in turn to see if the pupils react.
2) Touching a swab to the cornea, the transparent front 'window' of each eye, to see if it causes blinking.
3) Irrigating each ear in turn with a small volume of cold water to see if it causes movement of the eyes.
4) Passing a suction catheter into the windpipe to see if the patient gags or coughs.
5) Exerting pressure on the bony margin above the eye to see if the patient grimaces in response to pain.

If any one of these reflexes is present, it means that a part of the brainstem is still working and the tests are discontinued. However, if none of the brainstem reflexes can be stimulated, the two doctors apply what is known as the apnoea test: the ventilator is disconnected for a few minutes to see if the patient begins to breathe spontaneously. If movements of the chest wall are seen, testing is stopped. If not, the ventilator is reconnected until a second set of brainstem death tests is carried out, usually within a few hours. This second set of tests – identical to the first – serves as an additional safeguard for the patient.

When the second set of tests confirms the diagnosis of brainstem death, the ventilator is switched off. Or, if organ donation has been agreed, ventilation is continued until the organs are removed in the operating theatre. In either case, the formal time of death is that at which the first set of tests is completed.

Appendix II

Transplant Centres in the UK and Eire

Belfast	City Hospital	K
Birmingham	Queen Elizabeth Hospital	K, H, Li, Lu
	Diana, Princess of Wales Children's Hospital	Li
Bristol	Southmead Hospital	K
Cambridge	Addenbrooke's Hospital	K, Li, P
Cardiff	University Hospital of Wales	K, P
Coventry	University Hospital	K
Dublin	Beaumont Hospital	K
	St Vincent's Hospital	Li
	Mater Misericordiae Hospital	H, Lu
Edinburgh	Royal Infirmary	K, Li, P
Glasgow	Western Infirmary	K
	Golden Jubilee National Hospital	H
Harefield, Middlesex	Harefield Hospital	H, Lu
Leeds	St James's University Hospital	K, Li
Leicester	General Hospital	K

Liverpool	Royal Liverpool University Hospital	K
London	Great Ormond Street Hospital	K, H, Lu
	Guy's Hospital	K, P
	King's College Hospital	Li
	St George's Hospital	K
	The Royal Free Hospital	K, Li
	The Royal London Hospital	K
	W. London Renal and Transplant Centre	K, P
Manchester	Royal Infirmary	K, P
	Wythenshawe Hospital	H, Lu
Newcastle	Freeman Hospital	K, P, H, Li, Lu
Nottingham	City Hospital	K
Oxford	Churchill Hospital	K, P
Papworth Everard	Papworth Hospital	H, Lu
Plymouth	Derriford Hospital	K
Portsmouth	Queen Alexandra Hospital	K
Sheffield	Northern General Hospital	K

Key: K=kidneys, H=heart, Li=liver, Lu=lung, P=Pancreas

Source: NHSBT

Useful Organisations

AIH Support Group

16 Station Road, Lingwood, Norwich, Norfolk NR13 4AU; tel: 0845 3700 997. A website providing 'good quality information' in plain English on the liver condition autoimmune hepatitis
<http://www.autoimmunehepatitis.co.uk>

British Heart Foundation

Greater London House, 180 Hampstead Road, London NW1 7AW; tel: 0207 554 0000. Founded in 1961 by a group of clinicians concerned at the increasing death rate from cardiovascular disease. Provides information and support for patients, pioneers and funds research and lobbies for policies which reduce the risk of developing heart disease
<http://www.bhf.org.uk>

British Kidney Patient Association

2 The Windmills, St Mary's Close, Turk Street, Alton, Hants GU34 1EF; tel: 01420 541424. Set up in 1975 by Elizabeth Ward, the mother of a kidney patient, the BKPA soon came to spearhead a powerful lobby for kidney patients nationwide. Provides all-round support for kidney patients and their families and helps fund better services
<http://www.britishkidneypa-.co.uk>

British Liver Trust
2 Southampton Road, Ringwood, Hants BH24 1HY; tel: 01425 481320. The BLT is a national organisation, established in 1991, which offers help, information and support to people with liver or biliary disease, as well as to their families and carers/friends. The Trust also backs research and seeks to educate both healthcare personnel and the general public on matters relating to the liver <http://www.britishlivertrust.org.uk>

British Lung Foundation
73–75 Goswell Road, London EC1V 7ER; tel: 0207 688 5555. Established in 1985 and still the only charity working for everyone affected by lung disease. Provides information and support for patients and families and also funds world class research <http://www.lunguk.org>

British Transplantation Society
Chester House, 68 Chestergate, Macclesfield, Cheshire SK11 6DY; tel: 01625 664547. Established in 1972 to advance the study of issues relating to transplantation, to facilitate contact between people in the field and to disseminate knowledge <http://www.bts.org.uk>

Cardiomyopathy Association
Unit 10, Chiltern Court, Asheridge Road, Chesham, Bucks HP5 2PX; tel: 01494 791224. Founded in 1989, the Association helps patients with disorders of the heart muscle, provides information, funds specialist nursing posts and contributes to medical education <http://www.cardiomyopathy.org>

Child Death Helpline

Tel: 0800 282 986. Bereavement support service run jointly by two leading children's hospitals, London's Great Ormond Street and Alder Hey in Liverpool. Aiming to serve all those affected by the death of a child (no matter what the circumstances or when the death took place), it is manned by experienced volunteers, virtually all of whom are themselves bereaved parents
<http://www.childdeathhelpline.org.uk>

Children's Liver Disease Foundation

36 Great Charles Street, Queensway, Birmingham B3 3JY; tel: 0121 212 3839. The only charity concerned with all liver diseases in children, CLDF is active in education, research and emotional support for children, teenagers and families. It also spearheads initiatives to highlight the need for early recognition of paediatric liver problems
http://www.childliverdisease.org>

Compassionate Friends, The (TCF)

53 North Street, Bristol BS3 1EN; tel: 0845 120 3785. A nationwide organisation of bereaved parents, pioneered by a hospital chaplain in 1969, TCF offers help through 'befriending as distinct from counselling'. Membership open to all parents who have lost a child at any age and from any cause; special groups for parents of murdered children, child suicides and bereaved siblings
<http://www.tcf.org.uk>

Cruse Bereavement Care

PO Box 800, Richmond, Surrey TW9 1RG; tel: 0208 939 9530. Established in 1959, this is the UK's largest bereavement organisation, with branches throughout the British Isles. Cruse offers help to all bereaved people, regardless of age, circumstances, colour or creed. Also runs training courses for volunteers and healthcare personnel
http://www.crusebereavementcare.org.uk>

Cystic Fibrosis Trust

11 London Road, Bromley, Kent BR1 1BY; tel: 0208 464 7211. The CF Trust has been active for more than four decades on behalf of families affected by what is the UK's most common inherited disease (at time of going to print, affecting more than 9,000 people). It has been drawn into the transplantation arena with the development of lung transplantation and also owing to the appearance of terminal liver disease as a late complication of CF. The Trust funds a great many research projects <http://www.cftrust.org.uk>

Diabetes UK

Macleod House, 10 Parkway, London NW1 7AA; tel: 0207 424 1000. This is the UK's largest organisation working for people with diabetes, with more than 150,000 members at the time of going to print. Offers practical help, information and advice and reckons to spend almost £6 million a year on research <http://www.diabetes.org.uk>

Donor Family Network, The

PO Box 13825, Birmingham B42 9DJ; helpline: 0845 680 1954. Pioneered originally by one of the local transplant co-ordinators but now run by a donor parent, the network exists to support donor families and to promote organ donation. The network operates a donor quilt scheme to which families can contribute in memory of an organ donor <http://www.donorfamilynetwork.co.uk>

Heart Research UK

Suite 12D, Joseph's Well, Leeds LS3 1AB; tel: 0113 234 7474. Set up by a heart surgeon in 1967, HRUK financed six of the earliest UK heart transplants and has funded many

	research projects and community-based initiatives to help tackle heart disease <http://www.heartresearch.org.uk>
Hepatitis B Foundation UK	The Great Barn, Godmersham Park, Canterbury, Kent CT4 7DT; tel: 01227 738279. Set up in 2006, this charity seeks to draw together people with hepatitis B to give them a bigger collective voice, to enable support and to campaign for better services <http://www.hepb.org.uk>
Hepatitis C Trust, The	27 Crosby Row, London SE1 3YD; tel: 0207 089 6220. The Trust was set up in 2001 as a patient-led organisation to raise public awareness of hepatitis C, to counter discrimination and to provide information and support where needed <http://www.hepctrust.org.uk>
Human Tissue Authority, The	151 Buckingham Palace Road, London SW1W 9SZ; tel: 0207 269 1900. Formed to implement the Human Tissue Act 2004, the HTA is the regulatory body for all matters concerning the removal and retention of human tissue for transplantation, research or exhibition <http://www.hta.gov.uk>
Irish Kidney Association	Donor House, Block 43A, Park West, Dublin 12; tel: (353) 1620 5306. Established in 1978, the Association seeks to provide all-round care and support for kidney patients, including, in some cases, underwriting their care until it can be taken over by public funding <http://www.ika.ie>
Kidney Research UK	Nene Hall, Lynch Wood Park, Peterborough PE2 6FZ; tel: 0845 070 7601. This is a national charity funding research on the prevention, treatment and management of kidney disease <http://www.kidneyresearchuk.org>

Kidney Wales Foundation (KWF)

1 Radnor Court, 256 Cowbridge Road East, Cardiff CF5 1GZ; tel: 02920 343940. With a history dating back to 1967, KWF raises funds for and awareness of kidney patient care and research in Wales. It has contributed to some staff costs and, in 1986, was instrumental in setting up the computerised register known as Lifeline Wales for those willing to donate organs <http://www.kidneywales.com>

Legacy of Life

The Baker's Chest, Hartburn, Morpeth NE61 4JB. Run by a small group whose lives have been touched by transplantation, this charity was launched in 2006 to campaign for organ donation. The site features the illustrated book *Transforming Lives*, which relates personal stories of recipients and their families and of those who care for them <http://www.legacyoflife.org.uk>

Live Life then Give Life

PO Box 583, Epsom, Surrey KT17 9HD; tel: 0203 287 5595. Campaign launched in March 2006 by two young women, both suffering from cystic fibrosis, who between them had lost fifteen young friends awaiting transplants. The main thrust is to boost organ donation by encouraging people to sign up to the ODR and their team has organised media campaigns and a number of public events. Aims are to educate the public and give a voice to those affected by transplants and to offer them support <http://www.lltgl.org.uk>

National Kidney Federation	The Point, Coach Road, Shireoaks, Worksop, Notts S81 8BW; tel: 01909 544999. The only UK national charity run by kidney patients for kidney patients, it campaigns for a better deal for members, educates non-specialist doctors in up-to-the-minute treatments for renal disease, raises funds and backs research. Activities include purchase of medical equipment, provision of holiday facilities and help for patients and their families <http://www.kidney.org.uk>
NHS Blood and Transplant	NHSBT was set up as a special health authority in 2005, with responsibility for optimising the supply of blood, other tissues and organs and for raising the quality and effectiveness of transfusion and transplantation services. Its remit includes responsibility for the Organ Donation and Transplantation Directorate (formerly UK Transplant), whose functions include ensuring that donated organs are matched and fairly allocated. ODT campaigns to improve organ donation rates and maintains the NHS ODR (see below). The Directorate is based at Fox Den Road, Stoke Gifford, Bristol BS34 8RR; tel: 0117 975 7575 <http://www.organdonation.nhs.uk>
NHS Organ Donor Register	Introduced in autumn 1994, this is a computerised service enabling members of the public to record a willingness to donate their organs in the event of death. The register is run by the Organ Donation and Transplantation Directorate and can be contacted by ringing the Organ Donor Line: 0300 123 23 23.

Northern Ireland Transplant Association (NITA)	Eagle Lodge, 51 Circular Road, Belfast BT4 2GA; tel: 028 9076 1394. Run by a committee of volunteers, NITA is concerned with the support of people becoming involved with transplantation, whether on the recipient or donor side. It is also a source of information and works to promote organ donation <http://www.nitransplant.org>
PBC Foundation	54 Queen Street, Edinburgh EH2 3NS; tel: 0131 225 8586. The Foundation represents the interests of anyone affected by primary biliary cirrhosis, an autoimmune disease which may lead ultimately to liver failure. As well as supporting patients, together with their family and friends, it backs a number of research projects <http://www.pbcfoundation.org.uk>
PKD Charity, The	Foxhill Close, Langwith Road, Scarcliffe, Swansea SA4 6TH; tel: 0300 111 1234. Set up in 2001 as the only charity in the UK dedicated to providing information, advice and support to those affected by polycystic kidney disease, an inherited condition which is a common cause of kidney failure. Also funds research into the causes and treatment of PKD <http://www.pkdcharity.org.uk>
Save5	This is a one-woman campaign to persuade as many people as possible to sign up to the Organ Donor Register, the name reflecting the fact that the organs from one donor can save five lives. Diagnosed with not just one but two serious lung diseases in January 2010, T. Sandeman-Charles pioneered Save5

two months later, commissioned a website and set out as a public speaker with a personal target of securing 10,000 names for the ODR. <http://www.save5.org.uk>

To Transplant and Beyond

88 Woodthorpe Road, Ashford, Middlesex TW15 3JY; tel: 07956 312298. Charity established in 2000 by a heart transplant recipient in order to give support to other transplant patients and their families. Seeks to convey the positive side of transplantation as well as encouraging organ donation <http://www.heart-transplant.co.uk>

Transplant Sport UK

Basepoint Business Centre, 1 Winnall Valley Road, Winchester, Hants SO23 0LD; tel: 01962 832770. Established in 1978 following the first Transplant Olympics, the TSUK's main aim is to raise awareness of the need for organ donation. It does this by organising sporting and social events, including the annual British Transplant Games, to demonstrate the benefits of transplantation <http://www.transplantsport.org.uk>

Transplant Support Network, The

6 Kings Meadow Drive, Wetherby, West Yorkshire LS22 7FS; tel: 01937 585434. This is a nationwide network, pioneered in 1994, of volunteers – recipients and their carers – who provide support and reassurance to other patients, relatives and friends <http://www.transplantsupportnetwork.org.uk>

Welsh Kidney Patients' Association

Pentwyn Dialysis Unit, Unit 3, Avenue Industrial Estate, Croescardan Close, Pentwyn, Cardiff CF23 8HE; tel: 029 2074 2735. Established in 1982, the WKPA operates as a non-fundraising charity. It provides information and support, publishes its own magazine and runs the only independent patients' renal website in Wales. It also maintains a members' welfare fund <http://www.wkpa.org.uk>

Index